Research for
the Public Good

BRONFENBRENNER SERIES ON THE ECOLOGY
OF HUMAN DEVELOPMENT

Chaos and Its Influence on Children's Development: An Ecological Perspective
Edited by Gary W. Evans and Theodore D. Wachs

*Research for the Public Good: Applying the Methods of Translational Research to
    Improve Human Health and Well-Being*
Edited by Elaine Wethington and Rachel E. Dunifon

Research for the Public Good

Applying the Methods of Translational Research to Improve Human Health and Well-Being

EDITED BY
Elaine Wethington and Rachel E. Dunifon

AMERICAN PSYCHOLOGICAL ASSOCIATION
WASHINGTON, DC

Published by
American Psychological Association
750 First Street, NE
Washington, DC 20002
www.apa.org

To order
APA Order Department
P.O. Box 92984
Washington, DC 20090-2984
Tel: (800) 374-2721; Direct: (202) 336-5510
Fax: (202) 336-5502; TDD/TTY: (202) 336-6123
Online: www.apa.org/pubs/books
E-mail: order@apa.org

In the U.K., Europe, Africa, and the Middle East, copies may be ordered from
American Psychological Association
3 Henrietta Street
Covent Garden, London
WC2E 8LU England

Typeset in Goudy by Circle Graphics, Inc., Columbia, MD

Printer: United Book Press, Inc., Baltimore, MD
Cover Designer: Berg Design, Albany, NY

The opinions and statements published are the responsibility of the authors, and such opinions and statements do not necessarily represent the policies of the American Psychological Association.

Library of Congress Cataloging-in-Publication Data

Research for the public good : applying the methods of translational research to improve human health and well-being / edited by Elaine Wethington and Rachel E. Dunifon. — 1st ed.
    p. cm. — (APA Bronfenbrenner series on the ecology of human development)
    Includes index.
    ISBN 978-1-4338-1168-5 — ISBN 1-4338-1168-5 1. Medical care—Research. 2. Medical policy—Evaluation. 3. Medicine, Preventive. 4. Health—Social aspects. I. Wethington, Elaine. II. Dunifon, Rachel E. (Rachel Elizabeth)
    RA394.R47 2012
    362.1072—dc23

                                    2012007276

British Library Cataloguing-in-Publication Data

A CIP record is available from the British Library.

Printed in the United States of America
First Edition

DOI: 10.1037/13744-000

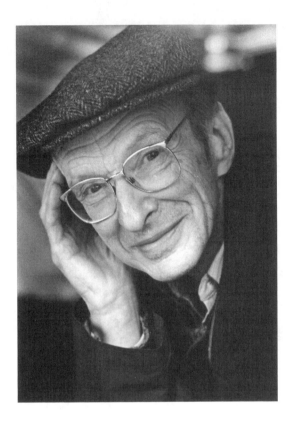

This series is dedicated to the personal memories and lasting theoretical insights of our friend, colleague, and mentor, Urie Bronfenbrenner. His thinking about human development has profoundly influenced so many students and colleagues in multiple areas of enquiry. We hope this series will provide another vehicle through which Urie's ideas on the bioecology of human development can continue to flourish.

This one is for "the Cletes."
—*Elaine Wethington*

To John, Jimmy, and Will—the light of my life.
—*Rachel "Red" E. Dunifon*

CONTENTS

CONTRIBUTORS

David M. Almeida, PhD, Professor, Department of Human Development and Family Studies, The Pennsylvania State University, University Park

Charles J. Brainerd, PhD, Professor, Department of Human Development, Cornell University, Ithaca, NY

Robert Crosnoe, PhD, Elsie and Stanley E. (Skinny) Adams, Sr. Centennial Professor of Liberal Arts, Departments of Sociology and Psychology, University of Texas at Austin

Ann C. Crouter, PhD, Dean, College of Health and Human Development; Professor of Human Development, Department of Human Development and Family Studies, The Pennsylvania State University, University Park

Kelly D. Davis, PhD, Research Assistant Professor, Department of Human Development and Family Studies, The Pennsylvania State University, University Park

Rachel E. Dunifon, PhD, Associate Professor, Director of Graduate Studies, and Department Extension Leader, Department of Policy Analysis and Management, Cornell University, Ithaca, NY

V. Jeffery Evans, MD, PhD, Director of Intergenerational Research (retired), Demographic and Behavioral Sciences Branch, The Eunice Kennedy Shriver National Institute for Child Health and Human Development, Bethesda, MD

Helena Herman, undergraduate student, Department of Human Development, Cornell University, Ithaca, NY

Jean M. Ispa, PhD, Professor and Cochair, Department of Human Development and Family Studies, University of Missouri, Columbia

Kimberly A. Kopko, PhD, Extension Associate, Department of Policy Analysis and Management, Cornell University, Ithaca, NY

Ludmila N. Krivitsky, BS, Research Assistant, Division of Geriatrics and Gerontology, Weill Cornell Medical College, New York, NY

Catherine A. Lesesne, PhD, MPH, Technical Director, Public Health Division, ICF Macro, Atlanta, GA

Rhoda Meador, Director, Gerontology Institute, Ithaca College, Ithaca, NY

Leigh Meckler, Intern, Division of Geriatrics and Gerontology, Weill Cornell Medical College, New York, NY

John W. O'Neill, PhD, Director, School of Hospitality Management, The Pennsylvania State University, University Park

Anusmiriti Pal, MD, Research Assistant, Division of Geriatrics and Gerontology, Weill Cornell Medical College, New York, NY

Samantha J. Parker, AB, Project Coordinator, Division of Geriatrics and Gerontology, Weill Cornell Medical College, New York, NY

Karl Pillemer, PhD, Hazel E. Reed Professor, Department of Human Development, Cornell University, Ithaca, NY; Professor of Gerontology in Medicine, Division of Geriatrics and Gerontology, Weill Cornell Medical College, New York, NY

M. Carrington Reid, MD, PhD, Joachim Silberman Family Clinical Scholar in Geriatric Palliative Care and Associate Professor of Medicine, Division of Geriatrics and Gerontology, Weill Cornell Medical College, New York, NY

Valerie F. Reyna, PhD, Codirector, Center for Behavioral Economics and Decision Research; Professor, Departments of Human Development, Psychology, Cognitive Science, and Neuroscience (IMAGINE Program), Cornell University, Ithaca, NY

Rouzi Shengelia, MD, Research Coordinator, Division of Geriatrics and Gerontology, Department of Medicine, Weill Cornell Medical College, New York, NY

Abraham H. Wandersman, PhD, Professor, Department of Psychology, University of South Carolina, Columbia

Elaine Wethington, PhD, Professor, Departments of Human Development and Sociology, Cornell University, Ithaca, NY

Eric Zember, graduate student, Human Development, Cornell University, Ithaca, NY

PREFACE

This volume, the second in the American Psychological Association (APA) Bronfenbrenner Series on the Ecology of Human Development, traces its inspiration to Urie Bronfenbrenner's 1996 book, *The State of Americans: This Generation and the Next*, coauthored with Peter McClelland, Elaine Wethington, Phyllis Moen, and Stephen Ceci. That book presented a compilation of statistics on crime, poverty, family well-being, education, and the like, with the goal of using "hard facts" to translate social scientific insight into a form that would influence policy and practice. One assumption of the book was that the adoption of practices and policies based on scientific evidence would improve the well-being of Americans. A second assumption was that social scientists should be at the table with policymakers in solving practical social problems and that research, to have high impact, must include practical implications for the improvement of health and development in the population. In essence, Bronfenbrenner and colleagues were promoting "translational research" without using the term.

The State of Americans exemplifies Bronfenbrenner's lifelong dedication to using research to improve the well-being of children and families. Bronfenbrenner, a developmental psychologist, rejected the idea of research for research's sake. As his life's major work, he developed a series of influential ecological theories related to human development, paying particular attention to the different contexts in which human development takes place—at the individual, family, institutional, and societal levels. At the heart of his theories and research was the interplay between people and their environment (person, process, context, and time). Bronfenbrenner took these innovations in theory and the research they inspired and sought to apply them—translate them—into meaningful implications for policy and practice. He sought not only to highlight the implications of his work but also to communicate his findings to policymakers and practitioners in effective ways. A key example of Bronfenbrenner's successful research translation was the active role he played in the founding of the Head Start program. In recognition of his lifetime contributions to applied psychology and to understanding critical social problems, Bronfenbrenner received the James McKeen Catell Fellow Award from the American Psychological Society (now the Association for Psychological Science) in 1993. In 1996, the APA Award for Lifetime Contribution to Developmental Psychology in the Service of Science and Society Award was renamed, in honor of Bronfenbrenner, the Urie Bronfenbrenner Award for Lifetime Contribution to Developmental Psychology in the Service of Science and Society.

The current volume emerges at a key time in the tradition of translational research. Fifteen years after the publication of *The State of Americans*, translational research has been promoted and funded by the National Institutes of Health, the Centers for Disease Control and Prevention, medical centers, and university programs as a means of speeding the application of basic science to the improvement of human health. We have realized Bronfenbrenner's vision from decades ago—using our best skills and research to improve the "state of Americans." We hope that this volume will encourage young researchers in the social and behavioral sciences to develop careers that help bridge the gaps among research, policy, practice, and the health and well-being of Americans. Contributors to this volume include experts in psychology, child development, public policy, sociology, gerontology, geriatric medicine, and economics; they discuss the concept of translational research, develop methods for translation of basic social and behavioral research into practice, and present case studies of translational research that have been led by social and behavioral scientists.

The chapters are based on papers prepared for a conference held to honor Bronfenbrenner on the Cornell University campus. The conference was sponsored by Cornell University's Bronfenbrenner Life Course Center and Cornell University's Family Life Development Center, which have subsequently merged to become the Bronfenbrenner Center for Translational Research (BCTR). The mission of BCTR is to build on and expand existing efforts by the College of Human Ecology and Cornell University to extend research-based knowledge into practice and policy settings. We are grateful to our colleagues who attended the conference and engaged in lively and informative discussion on the methods of translational research and the roles that social and behavioral scientists could play in such research. This volume attempts to capture their many insights and suggestions.

We are grateful to the expert reviewers who carefully critiqued each of the substantive chapters of this volume. We also wish to acknowledge the financial support of BCTR and Cornell University's College of Human Ecology, Institute for the Social Sciences, and Cooperative Extension. We give our deepest thanks to Carrie Chalmers, who handled organizational tasks for this book. Thanks are due to Maureen Adams and Beth Hatch for their patience as we edited drafts of the chapters. Thanks are also due to the editorial advisory committee for the series: Stephen J. Ceci, Gary W. Evans, Daniel Lichter, Karl Pillemer, Valerie F. Reyna, and Elaine Wethington.

Research for
the Public Good

INTRODUCTION: TRANSLATIONAL RESEARCH IN THE SOCIAL AND BEHAVIORAL SCIENCES

ELAINE WETHINGTON, HELENA HERMAN, AND KARL PILLEMER

Social and behavioral research is being used for the public good. To provide just one major example, Section 2951 of the Patient Protection and Affordable Care Act of 2010, better known as the "Health Care Reform Act," created a home visiting grant program for states. This program uses an evidence-based intervention model to improve the health and well-being of young mothers and their babies. Specifically, it uses the leading evidence-based home visiting model, the Nurse–Family Partnership, which was developed over the past 30 years by developmental psychologist David Olds through a series of randomized trials in three distinct and racially diverse geographical settings (Elmira, New York; Memphis, Tennessee; and Denver, Colorado). Currently, the Nurse–Family Partnership serves more than 20,000 young families in 20 states (Goodman, 2006).

This research was funded by an Edward R. Roybal Center Grant (1 P30 AG022845, Karl Pillemer and Mark Lachs, Principal Investigators); Grant2 P30 AG022845 (M. Carrington Reid and Karl Pillemer, Principal Investigators) from the National Institute on Aging; and an Interdisciplinary Geriatric Research Center grant from the John S. Hartford Foundation, administered by the RAND Corporation (M. Carrington Reid, Christopher S. Murtaugh, and Elaine Wethington, Principal Investigators). We thank Debra Goldman, Ethan Haymowitz, Ping-chun Liu, and Joran Seguira for their research assistance. We also thank Rachel E. Dunifon and Beth Hatch for their comments on this introduction.

The research that informed Section 2951 is one example of *translational research*, which is research linking scientific findings with programs and policies that improve human health and well-being. Translational research has been recognized as a significant priority by the National Institutes of Health (NIH) Office of Behavioral and Social Sciences Research (2007) in its Roadmap Initiative and by the current director (Collins, 2011). It has been promoted and funded by the NIH, the Centers for Disease Control and Prevention (CDC), medical centers, and university programs as a means of speeding the application of basic science to the improvement of human health.

The term *translational research* originally applied only to biomedical research that was used for disease prevention and treatment. In recent years, the definition has expanded to include physical, social, and behavioral research that is used for the improvement of human health and well-being. Applications of translational research include programs and policies involving education, disease prevention, health care delivery, health care access, and so forth.

Although translational research opportunities remain primarily biomedical and are housed in medical centers (Breckler, 2008; Perlstadt, 2009), opportunities for social and behavioral scientists to inform and take part in translational research are many and increasing. These opportunities include

- documenting individual factors (e.g., lifestyle, behavioral, decision making) that are associated with negative health and well-being outcomes;
- designing and demonstrating the efficacy of interventions to improve individual lifestyle, behavior, and decision making;
- creating academic–community networks to promote the use of evidence-based practices to improve community health and well-being;
- understanding diffusion of evidence-based programs through communities (e.g., social networks of researchers, practitioners, and consumers);
- developing a science of intervention adaptation and maintenance in the community;
- documenting social and health disparities and the community factors that are associated with widening or narrowing problematic disparities;
- understanding context-based factors that will have an impact on the success of interventions;
- adapting interventions to work effectively in racially and ethnically diverse communities;
- understanding and documenting the public health impact of wider community use of newly introduced evidence-based practices;

- influencing policymakers to promote the diffusion of evidence-based practices; and
- understanding the consequences, intended and unintended, of large interventions and policy changes.

This volume presents models and case studies illustrating the potential of translational research in the social and behavioral sciences. The overall goal is to generate insights that will guide the practice of translational research in the social and behavioral sciences and encourage researchers to develop careers that help bridge the gaps among research, policy, practice, and the health and well-being of Americans.

This introduction provides an overview of translational research and this volume. First, we analyze the history of the concept, including the varying definitions that have been promoted over the past decade. Definitions of translational research are important because they directly affect how social and behavioral sciences are included in the funding of such research. Next, we discuss methods for integrating social and behavioral sciences into translational research. Finally, we discuss the content and organization of this volume.

A BRIEF HISTORY OF THE CONCEPT OF TRANSLATIONAL RESEARCH

To some extent, it makes sense to discuss the history of translational research in two separate contexts, the medical research context and the social and behavioral research context. The two professional communities have historically had little interaction, with the findings from one having minimal influence on the activities of the other. As a result, the concept largely evolved separately in the two literatures.

Formulations in the Medical Literature

Concepts similar to *translation, translational science,* and *translational medicine* have been evident in the medical literature since the 1970s (for historical perspectives, see Drolet & Lorenzi, 2011; Perlstadt, 2009). Translational methods were promoted in cancer research in Great Britain and the United States through the NIH's National Cancer Institute and in research on HIV prevention (see Perlstadt, 2009). In these original formulations of translational research, social and behavioral sciences were explicitly included as a way of understanding the processes of transforming basic scientific findings into human interventions and evaluating the impact on public health

(Perlstadt, 2009). For example, in 2000, the National Institute of Mental Health (NIMH) formally highlighted the role of social and behavioral sciences in translational research when it issued a call for the translation of social and behavioral science into the diagnosis, prevention, and treatment of mental illness, leading to the funding of several translational research centers in the behavioral sciences (Perlstadt, 2009).

Although this early conceptualization of translational research included the social and behavioral sciences, an exclusively biomedical translational research movement subsequently emerged. The impetus for this biomedical movement was the 2001 report from the Institute of Medicine (IOM), *Crossing the Quality Chasm: A New Health System for the 21st Century* (Institute of Medicine Committee on Quality of Health Care in America, 2001). This report documented the slow pace at which scientific findings have been applied to the development effective treatments for disease and general public benefit in the United States despite heavy investment in biomedical research. Following the publication of the IOM report, NIH Director Elias Zerhouni proposed the adoption of translational research in the 2003 Roadmap (Zerhouni, 2003, 2005, 2007) intended to revitalize biomedical clinical research in the United States.

In the NIH Roadmap, Zerhouni (2003) proposed two types of translation. *Translation 1* (T1) was defined as the use of basic biomedical discoveries in clinical applications. (This is sometimes referred to, in biomedical shorthand, as the "left side" of the translational continuum.) *Translation 2* (T2) was defined as research intended to speed up the application of the new evidence-based clinical practices to the improvement of community health. (This research is referred to as the "right side" of the translational continuum.) Subsequently, several NIH institutes adopted Zerhouni's (2003) phrase "the process of applying ideas, insights, and discoveries generated through basic scientific inquiry to the treatment or prevention of human disease," a definition widely disseminated through the scientific and medical literature ("Editorial: Lost in clinical translation," 2004). This phrase explicitly referenced the need for a formal continuum between the two types of translation (and was used, eventually, to encourage the inclusion of social and behavioral sciences; National Institutes of Health, 2008). Often this is quickly reframed as "from the bench to the bedside"—a phrase that emphasizes the biomedical or treatment aspects of the definition rather than prevention. This two-part definition is prominent in the stated goals of the NIH Clinical and Translational Science Centers. To date, NIH has funded 60 medical school–based centers to further the goals of translational research described in the NIH Roadmap. These centers are required to promote both T1 and T2 research, engage researchers across multiple disciplines (e.g., medicine, public health, nursing, social work, neuroscience), develop ways to incorporate findings from T2 research to redirect T1 research, and engage the community in medical research (Sampselle, Pienta, & Markel, 2010).

Researchers have critiqued the 2003 NIH definition for a variety of reasons. Some have argued that referring to T1 and T2 research—two very distinct types of translation—by the same name leads to confusion and ambiguity about what in fact constitutes translational research and the types of skills that researchers need to acquire to adopt translational approaches in their research programs (e.g., Pincus, 2009; Woolf, 2008). In addition, the NIH two-part definition for translational research does not explicitly refer to the full potential of the social and behavioral sciences to contribute to the broader health research enterprise. This point was made clearly by Breckler (2008) in his critique titled "The NIH Roadmap: Are Psychologists In or Out?" The NIH definition of T1 refers explicitly to biomedical discoveries only. T2 could be construed to include a host of distinct activities, which may or may not be explicitly social or behavioral in approach. Thus, according to the biomedical definition of translational research, social and behavioral science is relevant only to T2 research (the right side of the continuum; see also Burgio, 2010).

Since the development of the T1 and T2 terminology, there have been a number of influential reinterpretations and extensions of the biomedical definition of translational research. We summarize these extensions heuristically in Figure 1, which portrays a series of steps in translating biomedical findings to human health applications, then to clinical practice and other interventions, and finally to public health improvements, with feedback loops along the way.

In refining the original T1 and T2 definitions, Sung et al. (2003), writing on behalf of an IOM panel, used the T1-T2 terminology adopted in the NIH Roadmap but explicitly included improvements in public health as the ultimate end point of T2; Sung et al. also indicated that clinical science and knowledge should be translated into both "clinical practice and health decision-making" (p. 1279). The inclusion of "health decision-making" in

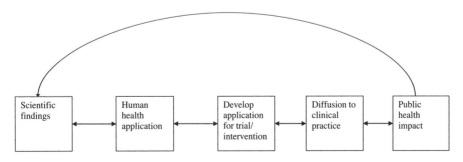

Figure 1. The evolving biomedical translational research model.

the definition of translational research thus includes clinicians and other health care professionals who prescribe treatments, the health care delivery system itself, industry, insurance companies, participants in clinical studies, and consumers of health care among the general public as target groups for translation (p. 1280). Under this more complex definition, T2 could range from research relating to effectiveness of treatments in different racial, ethnic, and social groups; to social and organizational barriers to the implementation of health interventions in clinical practices and communities; to consumer-based approaches to health; variations in health practice across cities, communities, and states; to dissemination of health innovations; and to health policy development. All of these research topics are in the purview of social and behavioral research.

Sung and colleagues (2003) also explicitly highlighted the bidirectional nature of influence between basic research and its applications. Among other suggestions, they recommended that barriers to participation in clinical research be addressed, particularly among minority groups; that clinical researchers acquire training to engage the public in research; and that the federal government increase its stake in health services and delivery research. Although Sung et al. conceived of translational research as primarily related to health conditions and treatment, they opened the door to collaboration with social and behavioral scientists having interest in health disparities and health care delivery systems. These groups include health and community psychologists, medical sociologists, health economists, and public policy scientists.

Sung's elaborated definition of T2 was broad, and many commentators have considered it unwieldy. Westfall, Mold, and Fagnan (2007) proposed a new category, *Translation 3* (T3), defined as "translation to practice" (as distinct from "translation to patients" or development of specific health treatments), dividing T2 into two categories (p. 405). They defined translational research as collaborative efforts by biomedical scientists and the larger community of public health and other service providers to apply evidence-based research ideas for improving overall population health (Westfall et al., 2007) rather than treatment of specific diseases and patients.

In defining the content of T3 research, Westfall et al. (2007) included some of the typical tools of social and behavioral science research as components of practice-based research, such as observational research and surveys, as well as applied social research on the means of implementation and dissemination to practice and communities. Another commentator addressing the broad nature of the T2 definition (Woolf, 2008) recommended that T2 be referred to by a label other than T1 because of the wide variety of research incorporated in it. Woolf (2008) asserted that T2 research is like T1 research "in name only" (p. 211) and that T2 requires researchers to have a very different set of research skills. Among such skills are those involving understanding the science of implementation in field and practice (see Fixsen, Naoom, Blase, Friedman, & Wallace, 2005); methods of evidence synthesis; epidemiology; communication and information systems; and theory including diffusions of innovations and dissemination (e.g., Glasgow, Lichtenstein, & Marcus, 2003; Rogers, 2003), social and psychological science (Burgio, 2010; Pillemer, Suitor, & Wethington, 2003), public policy, organizational science (e.g., McCall, 2009), and quality improvement and evaluation (Glasgow, Vogt, & Boles, 1999). Woolf also asserted that clinical settings were not the only settings in which translational research to improve health was relevant or where it could be developed; work settings and educational settings are also important consumers and disseminators of health information. Finally, he stated that the expanse of T2—"dissemination, health services, knowledge translation/transfer, implementation, or quality improvement" (p. 212)—was just as likely to be a major source for understanding health and disease as basic research in T1. Woolf's observations thus emphasized public health improvements as the ultimate outcome of translational research and (implicitly) the lessening of population health disparities (e.g., Wallerstein & Duran, 2010; Wallerstein, Yen, & Syme, 2011) as an important goal.

Similarly to Woolf and Sung and colleagues, Khoury et al. (2007) elaborated the translational continuum to include implementation, dissemination (or diffusion), outcomes research, and documentation of public health impact. Dougherty and Conway (2008) defined T3 as the "how" of delivering evidence-based, effective health care to the public to mitigate health disparities "so that evidence-based treatment, prevention, and other interventions are delivered reliably to all patients in all settings of care and improve the health of individuals and populations" (p. 2319). To previous lists of T2–T3 activities, they added studies of cost-effectiveness and health care redesign, in a continuous process of feedback to improve health care delivery. Drolet and Lorenzi (2011) argued that translational research (from T1 through T3) is a continuum that will also require implementation into public health programs as the end goal, through the implementation of practice-based research to assure that findings are put into practice. They noted that the process of translation "describes the transformation of knowledge through successive fields of research from a basic science discovery to public health" (pp. 1–2) through its impact on implementation, adoption, public health improvement, and a series of continuous feedback loops back to inspire more action.

In summary, elaborations of the translational continuum in the biomedical literature have come to focus on the types of contributions that social and behavioral scientists can make to multidisciplinary teams that aim to bridge gaps between different types of knowledge—specifically, moving evidence-based applications into wider use in health services and the community at large (NIH, 2008).

Formulations in the Social and Behavioral Science Literature

The term *translational research* was already being used in the social and behavioral sciences at the time it was adopted overall into the NIH Roadmap. Using a broad definition, Perlstadt (2009) argued that the field of sociology has been engaged in translational research for more than 100 years, applying sociological theories and findings to understanding and alleviating social problems. In addition, as noted earlier, social and behavioral scientists were funded by the NIMH and other NIH institutes to engage in translational research before the term was defined in the NIH Roadmap.

A case in point was a 2003 special issue of *The Gerontologist*, one of the journals published by the Gerontological Society of America. This issue was titled *Challenges of Translational Research on Aging: The Experience of the Roybal Centers*. The Edward R. Roybal Centers were established by the National Institute on Aging in 1993 to facilitate the translation of theory and basic research from the social and behavioral sciences into applied research, interventions, and programs to improve the quality of life, productivity, and health of older people. The Roybal Centers have been renewed every 5 to 6 years since 1993, with the latest reauthorization in 2009. In 2003, the Roybal Centers were refocused on "translational research on aging." A number of the Roybal Centers have been directed or codirected by social and behavioral scientists (Perlstadt, 2009), including psychologists, sociologists, and economists.

The 2003 special issue of *The Gerontologist* described a series of interventions and basic research projects executed by the early Roybal Centers, relating to mobility and driving, physical activity and falls prevention, exercise adherence, social integration into meaningful roles, cognition among aging patients with applications to medical settings, and technology use among older adults. In that issue, Pillemer et al. (2003) portrayed the translational research process as an application of social and behavioral science theory to intervention design and program development with the findings from the intervention then "translating back" for the development of better theory and—even more importantly—research more informed by the public and of demonstrated public health impact (p. 20). Also in this issue, Brown and Park (2003) described a process of using basic research on cognitive aging as a way to inform the development of new medical interventions and technologies for older patients. This was a model for translation to medical practice rooted in basic psychological research. (See also Cicchetti & Toth, 2009, for a model of translational research at the other end of the life span.)

Other articles in the special issue focused on how communication and social psychological theories could be applied to enhance motivation for health promotion (Farkas, Jette, Tennstedt, Haley, & Quinn, 2003) and how the application of ecological and systems design theories could improve research design (Czaja & Sharit, 2003). These articles predated the Zerhouni (2003) designation of T1 and T2, and none cited the 2001 IOM report. It could also be significant that none of these articles has been cited in the major biomedical reviews about the meaning and methods of translational research, perhaps indicating the height of the separate silos where biomedical and social science research findings tend to be stored.

METHODS FOR TRANSLATIONAL RESEARCH IN THE SOCIAL AND BEHAVIORAL SCIENCES

Along with other social scientists who have commented on the evolution of the translational research movement and opportunities for engaging social and behavioral scientists in translational activities (e.g., Breckler, 2008; Burgio, 2010; Krause, 2009), we believe that social and behavioral scientists can play a vital role in translational research. In Figure 2, we present a schema

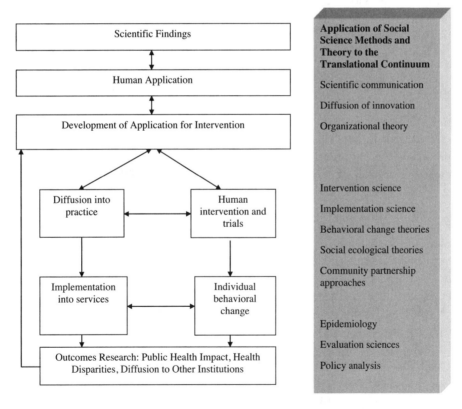

Figure 2. Application of social science theories and methods to translational research.

describing the how existing social science theories and methods can be incorporated into translational research. Specifically, we focus on how social and behavioral theories and methods can be used to bridge the "chasms" among the creation of basic scientific findings, application to humans, development of the application for human trials, diffusion into practice, creation of individual behavioral change, implementation into services, and impact on human health and well-being (see also NIH, 2008).

Theories of scientific communication, organizational theory, and diffusion of innovation (e.g., Rogers, 2003) are relevant in understanding how scientific communities can organize themselves to promote the application of basic scientific findings to humans (see Chapter 2, this volume). Social and behavioral intervention science (Burgio, 2010; Pillemer et al., 2003) and implementation science (e.g., Fixsen et al., 2005; see also Chapter 2, this volume) can be applied for designing human intervention and trials and for organizing and promoting diffusion to practitioners. Application of theories of behavioral change and social ecological theories in the social and behavioral sciences can be used to ensure that human intervention trials have an impact on individual behavior and lead to evidence that will promote implementation into services. Community partnership approaches (e.g., Israel, Schulz, Parker, & Becker, 1998) can be used to test the effectiveness of evidence-based interventions in diverse community groups (see Chapters 5, 6, and 8, this volume). The science of epidemiology, formal evaluation methods (e.g., RE-AIM, Glasgow et al., 1999), demography, and policy analysis methods apply to assessing population impact as well as to determining the need for interventions.

A specific social and behavioral science method that is being widely promoted for its applicability to translational research is community-based participatory research (CBPR). CBPR (Israel et al., 1998) is a partnership approach to research that involves community members, practitioners, and academic researchers equitably in all aspects of the research process, including conception of the research idea, planning, design of the research, implementation, evaluation, and dissemination of the findings. The aim of CBPR is to integrate research knowledge with practical on-the-ground knowledge and thereby increase the chances for new interventions and policy to succeed. CBPR is not a research method but an orientation toward research (Minkler & Wallerstein, 2003, p. 4). CBPR is also increasingly promoted as a way to improve the health of disadvantaged communities and promote health equity (Wallerstein & Duran, 2011). Penetration of CBPR into scientific health psychology has just begun, specifically through intervention design (Bogart & Uyeda, 2009), although it is already well established as a research orientation in community psychology, environmental psychology, and sociology (Krause, 2009).

CBPR has also been promoted as a way to foster interaction between universities and communities to bring research to bear on important social problems. For example, Carey et al. (2005) asserted that universities must collaborate with communities to gain the appropriate knowledge to understand and mitigate health disparities. They also emphasized that multidisciplinary research collaborations are necessary, drawing on medicine, epidemiology, social science, and economics to translate the findings of basic clinical and social science to local communities. Cargo and Mercer (2008) noted that the participatory approach is a way of engaging the community that can accommodate many types of designs and methods, including randomized controlled trials (e.g., Jernigan, 2010), as well as promoting the strength of existing communities to address issues of importance to the community, including health and health disparities.

The application of CBPR and other participatory research approaches (e.g., Jones & Wells, 2007) is not without controversy. Cargo and Mercer (2008) pointed out that the method has become a way to identify community health needs and interests and explore community-level behavioral risk factors and environmental conditions that are associated with poor health and means of effectively addressing behavioral risk factors in the local context, while engaging "the desire for other marginalized and underserved populations to assert control over the research and programs that affect them" (p. 330). They also pointed out that hard scientific evidence showing that participatory research methods are more effective than nonparticipatory research for community-based health studies is lacking (p. 340). Along with other commentators (e.g., Burgio, 2010), they called for research on the effectiveness of projects using participatory methods. We share Burgio's view but hope to demonstrate in this volume that partnership approaches at all levels and across disciplines are key in the translational research process.

ORGANIZATION OF THE VOLUME

The chapters in this volume are organized into two sections that relate to the key questions listed above: (a) social and behavioral science models for the translation of research; and (b) case studies showing how basic social and behavioral science can be translated into projects aimed at improving health, quality of life, and professional practice.

Section 1: Social and Behavioral Science Models for the Translation of Research

In Chapter 1, V. Jeffery Evans addresses how psychology and the other social and behavioral sciences can contribute to the effective translation of basic research to policy, practice, and overall quality of life. Evans discusses the recent development of translational research at NIH and how research priorities have been set to encourage the formation of multidisciplinary teams of medical, psychological, and behavioral scientists to address critical quality of life issues. These important issues include reducing health disparities, encouraging sustainable behavioral change, increasing the effectiveness of interventions, improving the dissemination of evidence-based practices, and engaging the community in research. Evans concludes by suggesting a model of translational research that can benefit both biomedical and social and behavioral science—one that takes into account the ways in which law and public policy influence translational research efforts.

In Chapter 2, Abraham H. Wandersman and Catherine A. Lesesne present a synthesis of research-to-practice models, discuss how the models relate to the different stages of translational research, and present ways to bridge the chasm between researchers and practice communities. They develop an original model, the Interactive Systems Framework, designed to improve research translation efforts for prevention in the community. This model focuses on bidirectional interactions between researchers and research "consumers" and argues that researchers need to become more informed about, and take into consideration, the needs and capacity of consumers to implement evidence-based programs.

In Chapter 3, Robert Crosnoe describes his use of research on learning to enhance understanding of inequalities in educational contexts and outcomes and, ultimately, to influence school and related public policies. Disparities in the educational system related to family socioeconomic circumstances, race, ethnicity, and immigration are important, timely policy issues that have a lifelong impact on health, health behavior, and social participation. A growing consensus in psychology, economics, and neuroscience holds that early childhood is a foundational period for the development of skills that carry youth into adulthood. Crosnoe's empirical studies of these issues, and his interdisciplinary approach, are a venue for understanding the two-way connection between research and policy and how researchers can increase their impact on policy. In this chapter, he describes his development as an interdisciplinary translational researcher through trial and error and comments on the lessons he has learned in translating basic research to policy applications and then back again while refining his approach to conducting science in partnership with community organizations.

In Chapter 4, a biomedical team based at Weill Cornell Medical College led by M. Carrington Reid presents a systematic analysis of research studies on adaptation of existing evidence-based programs to diverse communities and shows how raising standards for documentation and publication of such adaptation may advance the field and speed the process of research translation. Implementation of evidence-based programs is an important part of the translational research continuum (see Figure 2) and a marker of success. Evidence-based programs are those that have undergone formal evaluation using experimental or quasi-experimental methods. Entities such as CDC and NIH, however, recognize that programs may need to be adapted to improve fit for an individual organization, specifically to guarantee community participation across different situations and cultures. Important questions remain regarding how evidence-based programs can be adapted while preserving scientific effectiveness (Burgio, 2010). This chapter documents how program adaptation has been reported in the research literature, how well the adaptation has been documented, and whether the adaptation has followed strong scientific principles. The review concludes with recommendations for raising scientific standards for evidence-based program adaptations, including publication of guidelines by scientific societies, social and behavioral research on the implementation process itself, and higher standards for the application of theory in program adaptation.

Section 2: Four Case Studies for Translating Social and Behavioral Science to Improve Well-Being, Health, and Professional Practice

In Chapter 5, Jean M. Ispa describes concrete ways in which qualitative and quantitative research can be combined to better understand the impact of policy interventions and, ultimately, influence policymakers. An investigator in a program funded to evaluate Early Head Start programs across the country, Ispa describes how, by listening to the input of community educators, she discovered the value of taking a qualitative perspective when evaluating this important program. Among the advantages of using qualitative methods are the ability to shed light on local factors that influence program implementation and program effects and the production of findings that are accessible and interesting to all audiences. Ispa also comments on dilemmas that emerge in applying qualitative research, including ethical questions that come into play when observing the impacts of an intervention up close and personally, threats to research integrity, and management of power imbalances in relationships between researchers and study participants.

In Chapter 6, David M. Almeida, Kelly D. Davis, John W. O'Neill, and Ann C. Crouter report on their multilevel, multisite study of hotel employees and their families. This study is a collaboration of an interdisciplinary team of university-based investigators, hotel industry leaders, and hotel employees and their families. A major feature of the collaboration is that study findings have been incorporated into improving the science of measuring daily stress processes and the contagion of stressors into families and workplaces, with implications for improving workplace interventions to reduce absenteeism.

Almeida and coauthors describe a four-step process of translating information between the researchers and industry stakeholders, translating needs and concerns generated by the stakeholders into a study of daily life experiences, disseminating the findings to industry stakeholders, and applying the findings to design and evaluate a theoretically based but practical workplace intervention.

In Chapter 7, Eric Zember, Charles J. Brainerd, Valerie F. Reyna, and Kimberly A. Kopko describe a major success in the translation of basic psychological research to practice: the increasing influence of cognitive psychological findings about human mind and memory on the practice of law and the courts. As this chapter documents, cognitive psychologists have influenced practices of police interrogation, preparation of witnesses for trial, evaluation of the validity of eyewitness testimony, and practices assuring the credibility of child witnesses. The authors identify new research findings on memory, suggestibility, decision making, evaluation of risks, and neuroscience that they believe constitute the next frontier of translation of psychology to law and legal practices.

In Chapter 8, Elaine Wethington, Karl Pillemer, and Rhoda Meador describe their efforts to build an academic–practitioner partnership in New York City to facilitate rigorous, scientific research that addresses the concerns of front-line staff and directors of agencies and centers providing services to older people living in the five boroughs of New York. The aims of the partnership were to develop a communitywide set of research priorities, apply findings from social and behavioral sciences to practical issues threatening the well-being of older people, and speed the development of evidence-based practices and their implementation. To achieve these aims, the partnership created an innovative, multidisciplinary investigator development program to train researchers in the methods of translational research; an infrastructure to support researchers in the field; and a series of educational events for practitioners to increase their knowledge of research, research methods, and methods for dissemination of evidence-based practices by augmenting existing practitioner networks. A major lesson learned from the process is that partnerships across levels, professions, and disciplines are necessary in providing the support that investigators need to conduct translational research that has practical impact on the health of communities.

Finally, in Chapter 9, the editors summarize the major findings described in this volume and identify opportunities for increasing the contribution of psychological and other behavioral sciences to improving the quality of American life through collaboration in translational research. A major focus is on overcoming the challenges of conducting translational research: fostering productive collaboration across disciplines, ensuring effective adoption of evidence-based practices, and speeding the translation of basic scientific findings into practice and policy. A key finding emerging in this volume is the importance of partnerships across disciplines and between scientists and community stakeholders.

REFERENCES

Bogart, L. M., & Uyeda, K. (2009). Community-based participatory research: Partnering with communities for effective and sustainable behavioral health interventions. *Health Psychology, 28*, 391–393. doi:10.1037/a0016387

Breckler, S. J. (2008). The NIH Roadmap: Are psychologists in or out? *Journal of Clinical Psychology in Medical Settings, 15*, 60–64. doi:10.1007/s10880-008-9099-6

Brown, S., & Park, D. C. (2003). Theoretical models of cognitive aging and implications for translational research in medicine. *The Gerontologist, 43*(Suppl. 1), 57–67. doi: 10.1093/geront/43.suppl_1.57

Burgio, L. D. (2010). Disentangling the translational sciences: A social science perspective. *Research and Theory for Nursing Practice: An International Journal, 24*(1), 56–63. doi:10.1891/1541-6577.24.1.56

Carey, T. S., Howard, D. L., Goldman, M., Roberson, J. T., Godley, P. A., & Ammerman, A. (2005). Developing effective interuniversity partnerships and community-based research to address health disparities. *Academic Medicine, 80*(11), 103–1045. doi:10.1097/00001888-200511000-00012

Cargo, M., & Mercer, S. L. (2008). The value and challenges of participatory research: Strengthening its practice. *Annual Review of Public Health, 29*, 325–350. doi:10.1146/annurev.publhealth.29.091307.083824

Cicchetti, D., & Toth, S. L. (2009). The past achievements and future promises of developmental psychopathology: The coming of age of a discipline. *Journal of Child Psychology and Psychiatry, 50*(1–2), 16–25. doi:10.1111/j.1469-7610.2008.01979.x

Collins, F. S. (2011). Reengineering translational science: The time is right. *Science Translational Medicine, 3*(90), 90cm17. doi:10.1126/scitranslmed.3002747

Czaja, S. J., & Sharit, J. (2003). Practically relevant research: Capturing real world tasks, environments, and outcomes. *The Gerontologist, 43*(Suppl. 1), 9–18. doi: 10.1093/geront/43.suppl_1.9

Dougherty, D., & Conway, P. H. (2008). The "3T's" road map to transform US health care: The "how" of high-quality care. *JAMA, 299*, 2319–2321. doi:10.1001/jama.299.19.2319

Drolet, B. C., & Lorenzi, N. M. (2011). Translating research: Understanding the continuum from bench to bedside. *Translational Research, the Journal of Laboratory and Clinical Medicine, 157*, 1–5. doi:10.1016/j.trsl.2010.10.002

Editorial: Lost in clinical translation. (2004). *Nature Medicine, 10,* 879. doi:10.1038/ nm0904-879

Farkas, M., Jette, A. M., Tennstedt, S., Haley, S. M., & Quinn, V. (2003). Knowledge dissemination and utilization in gerontology: An organizing framework. *The Gerontologist, 43*(Suppl. 1), 47–56. doi: 10.1093/geront/43.suppl_1.47

Fixsen, D. L., Naoom, S. F., Blase, K. A., Friedman, R. M., & Wallace, F. (2005). *Implementation research: A synthesis of the literature.* Tampa, FL: University of South Florida, National Implementation Research Network.

Glasgow, R. E., Lichtenstein, E., & Marcus, A. C. (2003). Why don't we see more translation of health promotion research to practice? Rethinking the efficacy-to-effectiveness transition. *American Journal of Public Health, 93,* 1261–1267. doi:10.2105/AJPH.93.8.1261

Glasgow, R. E., Vogt, T. M., & Boles, S. M. (1999). Evaluating the public health impact of health promotion interventions: The RE-AIM framework. *American Journal of Public Health, 89,* 1322–1327. doi:10.2105/AJPH.89.9.1322

Goodman, A. (2006). *The story of David Olds and the Nurse Home Visiting Program.* Robert Wood Johnson Foundation. Retrieved from http://www.rwjf.org/files/ publications/other/DavidOldsSpecialReport0606.pdf

Institute of Medicine Committee on Quality of Health Care in America. (2001). *Crossing the quality chasm: A new health system for the 21st century.* Washington, DC: National Academies Press.

Israel, B. A., Schulz, A. J., Parker, E. A., & Becker, A. B. (1998). Review of community-based research: Assessing partnership approaches to improve public health. *Annual Review of Public Health, 19,* 173–202. doi:10.1146/annurev. publhealth.19.1.173

Jernigan, V. B. (2010). Community-based participatory research with Native American communities: The chronic disease self-management program. *Health Promotion Practice, 11*(6), 888–899. doi:10.1177/1524839909333374

Jones, L., & Wells, K. (2007). Strategies for academic and clinical engagement in community-participatory partnered research. *JAMA, 297,* 407–410. doi:10.1001/ jama.297.4.407

Khoury, M. J., Gwinn, M., Yoon, P. W., Dowling, N., Moore, C., & Bradley, L. (2007). The continuum of translation research in genomic medicine: How can we accelerate the appropriate integration of human genome discoveries into health care and disease prevention? *Genetics in Medicine, 9,* 665–674. doi:10.1097/ GIM.0b013e31815699d0

Krause, J. D. (2009). Taking it into the interactional field: Toward translational applied sociology. *Humboldt Journal of Social Relations, 32*(1), 35–85.

McCall, R. B. (2009). Evidence-based programming in the context of practice and policy. *SRCD Social Policy Report, 23*(3), 3–11.

Minkler, M., & Wallerstein, N. (Eds.). (2003). *Community-based participatory research for health.* San Francisco, CA: Jossey-Bass.

National Institutes of Health. (2008). *Request for information (RFI): Public comment on development of a funding opportunity announcement on translating discoveries in the basic behavioral and social sciences* (NIH Publication No. NOT-HL-08-114). Retrieved from http://grants.nih.gov/grants/guide/notice-files/NOT-HL-08-114.html

Office of Behavioral and Social Sciences Research. (2007). *The contributions of behavioral and social sciences research to improving the health of the nation: A prospectus for the future*. Washington, DC: U.S. Department of Health and Human Services, National Institutes of Health.

Perlstadt, H. (2009). Translational research: enabling the biomedical and social behavioral sciences to benefit society. *Humboldt Journal of Social Relations, 32*(1), 4–34.

Pillemer, K. A., Suitor, J. J., & Wethington, E. (2003). Integrating theory, basic research, and intervention: Two case studies from caregiving research. *The Gerontologist, 43*(Suppl. 1), 19–28. doi: 10.1093/geront/43.suppl_1.19

Pincus, H. A. (2009). Commentary: Challenges and pathways for translational research: Why is this research different from all other research? *Academic Medicine, 84*, 411–412. doi:10.1097/ACM.0b013e31819a8210

Rogers, E. M. (2003). *Diffusion of innovations* (5th ed.). New York, NY: Free Press.

Sampselle, C. M., Pienta, K. J., & Markel, D. S. (2010). The interdisciplinary and bidirectional mandate to accomplish translation. The CTSA mandate: Are we there yet? *Research and Theory for Nursing Practice: An International Journal, 24*(1), 64–73. doi:10.1891/1541-6577.24.1.64

Sung, N. S., Crowley, W. F., Genel, M., Salber, P., Sandy, L., Sherwood, L. M. . . . Rimoin, D. (2003). Central challenges facing the national clinical research enterprise. *JAMA, 289*, 1278–1287. doi:10.1001/jama.289.10.1278

Wallerstein, N., & Duran, B. (2011). Community-based participatory research contributions to intervention research: The intersection of science and practice to improve health equity. *American Journal of Public Health, 100*, S40–S46.

Wallerstein, N., Yen, I. H., & Syme, S. L. (2011). Integration of social epidemiology and community-engaged interventions to improve health equity. *American Journal of Public Health, 101*, 822–830. doi:10.2105/AJPH.2008.140988

Westfall, J. M., Mold, J., & Fagnan, L. (2007). Practice-based research—blue highways on the NIH Roadmap. *JAMA, 297*, 403–406. doi:10:1001/jama.297.4.403

Woolf, S. H. (2008). The meaning of translational research and why it matters. *JAMA, 299*, 211–213. doi:10.1001/jama.2007.26

Zerhouni, E. A. (2003, October 3). The NIH Roadmap. *Science, 302*, 63–72. doi:10.1126/science.1091867

Zerhouni, E. A. (2005). Translational and clinical science—time for a new vision. *The New England Journal of Medicine, 353*, 1621–1623. doi:10.1056/NEJMsb053723

Zerhouni, E. A. (2007). Translational research: Moving discovery to practice. *Clinical Pharmacology & Therapeutics, 81*, 126–128. doi:10.1038/sj.clpt.6100029

I

SOCIAL AND BEHAVIORAL SCIENCE MODELS FOR THE TRANSLATION OF RESEARCH

1

TRANSLATION IN THE SOCIAL AND BEHAVIORAL SCIENCES: LOOKING BACK AND LOOKING FORWARD

V. JEFFERY EVANS

What is *translation* in the social and behavioral sciences? At its core, translation means relating an insight from basic scientific investigation to something that is useful for promoting the well-being of one or more humans. As noted in the Introduction to this volume, the medical model of translation is often proposed as a standard to which the social and behavioral sciences should aspire. In this chapter, I argue that much is to be gained by adopting the medical model as a starting point for research translation in the social and behavioral sciences, as long as this model evolves to incorporate the complexities of the social environment in which research translation takes place. I discuss a unique model of translational research, particularly relevant to the behavioral and social sciences, which includes a consideration of the political, legal, and budgetary environment, and I argue that this new model can benefit the fields of both medicine and social and behavioral science.

DEFINITIONS OF TRANSLATIONAL RESEARCH

Currently, there is much emphasis at the National Institutes of Health (NIH) on translational research: NIH is the driving force of translation in medicine. Typically, translation has been expressed as it appeared in an NIH request for applications (RFA; RFA-AR-05-005), issued in 2005:

> Translational research is defined as applied and clinical scientific research that is directed towards testing the validity and limits of applicability of knowledge derived from basic science and engineering to the understanding of human diseases and health. It could be research involving living human subjects (i.e., clinical) but it might also be non-clinical involving the study of human genes, tissues, specimens, or cells. Thus, although it is directed towards generation of knowledge about humans, it could be non-clinical or clinical research. It could be knowledge useful to persons (individuals, families, and populations) affected by or at risk for specific diseases. (p. 2)

The medical model of translation focuses on moving knowledge from the laboratory to human application and then moving the application through a series of rigorous randomized controlled trials (RCTs) to medical practice or public health policy (e.g., Sung et al., 2003). At its core, the medical model asks the following questions: Can we apply a basic discovery to humans? Is the application safe for human use? How can humans best use the application?

However, the medical model has had to adjust to accommodate the considerations of external forces such as health care practice and policy. For example, in response to politically based concerns about the cost of health care, the concept of translational research in medicine now includes cost-effectiveness of applications as core elements. A 2008 RFA from the Eunice Kennedy Shriver National Institute of Child Health and Human Development (NICHD) captures this point (RFA-HD-08-008):

> Translational research includes two areas of translation. One is the process of applying discoveries generated during research in the laboratory, and in preclinical studies, to the development of trials and studies in humans. The second area of translation concerns research aimed at enhancing the adoption of best practices in the community. Cost-effectiveness of prevention and treatment strategies are also an important part of translational science. (NIH, 2008c, p. 2)

NICHD is the key agency home for human development research in NIH. Urie Bronfenbrenner's concepts of human development, in which individual development is influenced by a variety of factors at the family, neighborhood, school, and more macro levels, are part of the NICHD mission. Two extramural branches at NICHD incorporate Bronfenbrenner's model. The Child Development Branch looks at child development as Bronfenbrenner would, considering a variety of levels of influence on child development from the child's perspective. The Demographic and Behavioral Sciences Branch looks at children as a demographic group and examines the contextual influences on the group.

These two branches together recently initiated a program called the Science and Ecology of Development (NIH, 2008b), which expressly took Bronfenbrenner's perspective into account to explain the development of disadvantaged children. Given the way in which his model of child development has been incorporated into the NICHD funding structure, it is fair to ask whether Bronfenbrenner would be totally satisfied with the definition of translational research expressed in the two RFAs quoted above. I think not. Why? It lacks specific attention to law, public policy, and public expenditure. An ideal model for basic research in the social and behavioral sciences does more than encompass the common notion of translation in the medical world by focusing on speeding insights from basic science to improve clinical practice and facilitate basic research driven by the needs of clinical practice. It moves beyond that model to incorporate aspects that are relevant to both law and public policy.

LAW AND PUBLIC POLICY DIMENSIONS OF RESEARCH TRANSLATION

The law and public policy dimensions of social and behavioral research give rise to nuances of translation that extend the traditional medical concepts in directions that increase the relevance of both biomedical research on one hand and social, behavioral and psychological research on the other. These developments come just at the right time. Biomedical research now must confront major public policy initiatives in the area of health insurance reform and its requirement that we find collective ways of improving care while lowering its cost (see the Affordable Care Act, which is the Patient Protection and Affordable Care Act enacted on March 23, 2010, as amended by the Health Care and Education Reconciliation Act on March 30, 2010). At the same time, behavioral and social science research must now take a more medically based perspective and confront the role that human biology plays in behavioral responses to social incentives.

Where does this leave the question of defining translation? The traditional medical definition of translational research must be broadened to include useful knowledge from the social and behavioral sciences regarding health and human development at the individual, familial, population, and governmental levels. Inclusion of such knowledge improves not only clinical practice but also law and public policy. The new director of NIH, Francis Collins, embraced an enlarged concept of translation when he announced five major themes that would characterize his directorship, including an explicit acknowledgment of the role of public policy, when he emphasized putting "science to work for the benefit of health care reform" ("New NIH director," 2009). In doing so, Director Collins defined a translation concept that is quite serviceable for the needs of the social and behavioral sciences in that it incorporates an understanding of the political and social context in which translational research takes place.

Many scholars in the behavioral and social sciences encounter the translation question by doing *policy-relevant* research, which can be defined most generally as research that can help policymakers make plans, policies, and funding decisions. Examining this familiar concept in more detail can shed light on the process of research translation and how the meaning of such translation is changing. Typically, policy-relevant research tells us about how a law or policy changes human behavior or illuminates the need and opportunity to implement an effective law or policy. Usually such research has as its core a theory arising out of one of the constituent disciplines in the social and behavioral sciences. Research translation consists of an application of theories to illuminate a problem or solution of practical importance to law or public policy (see Chapter 7, this volume). This is the essence of applied research, and it becomes translation when such research is used to say something definitive about the need for or the effect of law and public policy. Such research can take many forms, from experimental studies in which human participants are randomly assigned to various policy regimes or programs, to descriptive studies that illuminate the context in which public policies or programs are being enacted, to longitudinal studies that examine how individuals exposed to various conditions change over time.

PROSPECTS FOR SOCIAL AND BEHAVIORAL RESEARCH TRANSLATION

The NIH community has been examining the basic social and behavioral research that it supports to see where NIH might stimulate the field to have the most impact on its core mission. The initiative is called the Science of Behavior Change (SOBC; see Rose Li and Associates, 2009). A large conference was held on the NIH campus on June 15–16, 2009, to brainstorm the opportunities and challenges facing NIH. One of them presents itself in the form of health care policy and the attempts to change it. There are basic and applied science dimensions to this issue, and the social, behavioral, and psychological research communities have a substantial role in both.

An idea that emerged in the NIH conference is the realization that biomedical translation often fails to scale up to effective population-level programs. A good example of this problem can be seen in the controversy concerning the safety of estrogen replacement therapy for the treatment of menopause. Evidence that accumulated from several randomized trials in the Women's Health Study (e.g., Writing Group for the Women's Health Initiative Investigators, 2002) conflicted with the findings of several large observational studies. It is now clear that we need findings from both types of studies to begin to make sense of such complex issues. This, of course, is an important consideration for health care reform, which is intended to be effective nationwide.

Thus, many in the NIH community see the need for a new a new type of methodology that links individual and community-level factors simultaneously and over time. They also see the need to address bundles of behaviors that are mutually reinforcing at the individual, family, and social network levels. This highlights the key role that social and behavioral science can play. Evidence-based medicine derived through RCTs is perceived as methodologically rigorous because it is definitive and concrete internally within a controlled experimental setting. However, the external validity of such research is less well known, and a greater understanding of the synergies among biology, individual contexts, families, networks and communities, and public policy is needed (e.g., Burgio, 2010). To address this need, NIH has set aside funds for interdisciplinary project-focused research that highlights the contexts in which healthy development occurs. This research includes the Opportunity Network (National Institutes of Health, 2010a) and the Economics of Health Care Reform (National Institutes of Health, 2010b). Projects funded under these mechanisms are designed to incubate important ideas that will enable many productive approaches to translation, including policy translation by putting the traditional medical model of translational research into a larger social and political context.

METHODS FOR SOCIAL AND BEHAVIORAL RESEARCH TRANSLATION

What methodology should be used by social, behavioral, and psychological sciences in conducting research relevant to policy translation? To answer this question, I start with the medical model, which relies on evidence-based methodology. As noted above, in biomedical science, the controlled experiment is king, and its manifestation in human clinical science is the RCT.

The policy research community shares this high regard for experimental design studies to validate policy effectiveness (e.g., Rittenhouse, Thom, & Schmittdiel, 2010). Armed with this approach we can say much about the efficacy, safety, and dosing of drugs, therapies, and even policy provisions. However, how can this knowledge help us understand complex political issues such as health care policy? Can such research help us understand the extent to which society will adopt, adhere to, and maintain efficient behaviors and therapies in the real world? Can it assure effective decision making in implementing complex health care systems? While the RCT approach can illuminate the numerous behavioral mechanisms and tendencies involved in these questions, it is less well equipped to illuminate how interventions or policy changes operate in the real world.

Social and behavioral sciences can provide critical data that may help bridge the gap from RCTs to policy. Such research can add a variety of observational data gathering and analytic techniques to experimental analyses to improve generalization and to account for biases that often creep into the best controlled studies. For example, social and behavioral science can be used to provide descriptive information on the community including family, social, or political context in which interventions or policies are taking place, shedding light on the contexts in which desired changes are more likely to occur and on instances in which change is more difficult. Moreover, through the use of rich, longitudinal data containing a wide range of social and psychological measures, social and behavioral science research can measure and shed light on the complicated pathways by which policies and interventions unfold over time. With the help of additional research such as that contemplated by SOBC, social and behavioral scientists can add much more to policy translation in regard to health care reform and myriad other policies as well. Combining experimental and observational techniques might even become the new gold standard in policy-relevant work.

NEW APPROACHES TO RESEARCH

Several social science data collection techniques deserve special mention in discussing translational research because they enhance realism and relevance in policy studies. Qualitative research can be combined with traditional quantitative research to form powerful combinations. When qualitative research is embedded in a quantitative study, the interaction of styles can increase the relevance and interpretation of the data and add dimensions to the analysis that are useful for policy translation (Shavelson & Towne, 2002; see also Chapter 5, this volume). Through the gathering of qualitative information, researchers can shed light on nuanced issues such as why some individuals take up programs or policies while others do not, how policies or programs are perceived by individuals and how that perception varies, and the conditions under which policy interventions are more likely to succeed.

Another approach, community-based participatory research (CBPR; Israel, Schulz, Parker & Becker, 1998; Wallerstein & Duran, 2010), requires that researchers create and maintain partnerships with communities of interest. In such a model, scientific investigation arises out of the interaction among partners (see Chapter 8, this volume). It is a way of focusing on the information and interventions that the community really wants to know about or engage. As such, successful data gathering or intervention research is well positioned to feed back into the community at a rapid rate. CBPR can aid research translation in two ways: It can identify policy-relevant information and it can help the research community relate helpful information back to stakeholders in the community of interest (Wallerstein & Duran, 2010). While CBPR is not a substitute for scientific measurement of communities or community processes, it is good at creating a sense of partnership with a community and for eliciting ideas and reactions to ideas that are the most relevant to communities. Scientific attempts to measure the community context whether it be in quantitative, qualitative, or mixed-method form, do not substitute for the development of community partnerships.

NIH has realized the significance of CBPR and now has a trans-NIH interest group organized to facilitate CBPR approaches into the mainstream of NIH funding processes. In so doing, NIH has organized two generations of funding announcements, which have featured specialized reviews designed to build experts on the CBPR process into the NIH peer review system (see PAR-08-075, NIH, 2008a). The recognition of the worth of CBPR research is a major milestone in the development of CBPR research and could signal an age in which the research community adds a new dimension to translational research in areas such as cancer (Hebert, Brandt, Armstead, Adams, & Steck, 2009).

SUMMARY AND CONCLUSION

The complex political and social policies being implemented today, such as health care reform, provide challenges for the basic research community. Specifically, translational research is needed that not only takes into account the medical model of RCTs but also incorporates insights from social and behavioral science that focus on the social and political contexts in which policy changes occur and the conditions and processes under which such changes succeed or fail.

It is apparent that all types of applied research—observational, longitudinal, and experimental—are useful in policy translation. It is also important to acknowledge that public policy is necessarily a process that requires frequent modification and innovation. The research community should not expect to formulate a policy innovation that will solve complex problems in one fell swoop. Rather, researchers should gird themselves to engage the public policy process and to translate both a factual critique of current policy and possible policy innovations as part of an ongoing relationship with policymakers. I had the opportunity to see Urie Bronfenbrenner in action as an adviser in federal policymaking, and it was clear that he understood this point. Bronfenbrenner would do great science and come to Washington and sit attentively in cramped meeting rooms, not leaving until he was understood.

NIH instituted a long-term initiative using the NIH director's common fund to provide grants for research dealing with numerous aspects of health care reform (see http://nihroadmap.nih.gov/healtheconomics/grants.asp). The basic science community has an important role in this new area of policy formulation. That role is to produce a comprehensive description of the hard facts pertaining to the problem of health care reform, insight into the ways in which health care reform can affect the health and welfare of Americans, and principles that may better evaluate the costs and benefits of reform. Bronfenbrenner would likely be eager to contribute to this domain in public policy because it means so much to families and children. I am confident that social and behavioral scientists will continue to contribute to Bronfenbrenner's legacy through their engagement in policy-relevant translational research on a variety of topics.

REFERENCES

Burgio, L. D. (2010). Disentangling the translational sciences: A social science perspective. *Research and Theory for Nursing Practice, 24*(1), 56–63. doi:10.1891/1541-6577.24.1.56

Hebert, J. R., Brandt, H. M., Armstead, C. A., Adams, S. A., & Steck, S. E. (2009). Interdisciplinary, translational, and community-based participatory research: Finding a common language to improve cancer research. *Cancer Epidemiology, Biomarkers & Prevention, 18*(4), 1213–1217. doi:10.1158/1055-9965.EPI-08-1166

Israel, B. A., Schulz, A. J., Parker, E. A., & Becker, A. B. (1998). Review of community-based research: Assessing partnership approaches to improve public health. *Annual Review of Public Health, 19*, 173–202. doi:10.1146/annurev.publhealth.19.1.173

National Institutes of Health. (2005). *Centers of research translation* (NIH Publication No. RFA-AR-05-005). Retrieved from http://grants.nih.gov/grants/guide/rfa-files/RFA-AR-05-005.html

National Institutes of Health. (2008a). *Community partnership research targeting the medically underserved (R01)* (NIH Publication No. PAR-08-075). Retrieved from http://grants.nih.gov/grants/guide/rfa-files/RFA-HD-08-075.html

National Institutes of Health. (2008b). *The science and ecology of human development (SEED) (R01)* (NIH Publication No. PA-08-069). Retrieved from http://grants.nih.gov/grants/guide/pa-files/PA-08-069.html

National Institutes of Health. (2008c). *Translational research on female pelvic floor disorders (R01)* (NIH Publication No. RFA-HD-08-008). Retrieved from http://grants.nih.gov/grants/guide/rfa-files/RFA-HD-08-008.html

National Institutes of Health. (2010a). *Effects of the social environment on health: Measurement, methods, and measures* (NIH Publication No. RFA-DA-11-003). Retrieved from http://grants.nih.gov/grants/guide/rfa-files/RFA-DA-11-003.html

National Institutes of Health. (2010b). *Science of structure, organization and practice design in the efficient delivery of effective healthcare (R21)* (NIH Publication No. RFA-RM-10-016). Retrieved from http://grants.nih.gov/grants/guide/rfa-files/RFA-RM-10-016.html

New NIH director Dr. Francis Collins on medical research that benefits everyone's health. (2006, Fall). *NIH MedlinePlus*. Retrieved from http://www.nlm.nih.gov/medlineplus/magazine/issues/fall09/articles/fall09pg2-4.html

Rittenhouse, D. R., Thom, D. H., & Schmittdiel, J. A. (2010). Developing a policy-relevant research agenda for the patient-centered medical home: A focus on outcomes. *Journal of General Internal Medicine, 25*, 593–600. doi:10.1007/s11606-010-1289-x

Rose Li and Associates. (2009). NIH Science of Behavior Change: Meeting summary. Retrieved from http://commonfund.nih.gov/documents/SOBC_Meeting_Summary 2009.pdf

Shavelson, R. J., & Towne, L. (2002). *Scientific research in education*. Washington, DC: National Academies Press.

Sung, N. S., Crowley, W. F., Genel, M., Salber, P., Sandy, L., Sherwood, L. M. . . . Rimoin, D. (2003). Central challenges facing the national clinical research enterprise. *JAMA, 289*, 1278–1287. doi:10.1001/jama.289.10.1278

Wallerstein, N., & Duran, B. (2010). Community-based participatory research contributions to intervention research: The intersection of science and practice to improve health equity. *American Journal of Public Health, 100*(S1), S40–S46. doi:10.2105/AJPH.2009.184036

Writing Group for the Women's Health Initiative Investigators. (2002). JAMA, *288*, 321–333. doi:10.1001/jama.288.3.321

2

IF TRANSLATIONAL RESEARCH IS THE ANSWER, WHAT'S THE QUESTION? WHO GETS TO ASK IT?

ABRAHAM H. WANDERSMAN AND CATHERINE A. LESESNE

With the need to address the spiraling costs of health care in the United States and around the world, funders such as the National Institutes of Health (NIH) and the Centers for Disease Control and Prevention (CDC) and scientists are placing more emphasis on translational research. After an idea or an intervention was described to Urie Bronfenbrenner, he often replied, "What's the question?" In other words: What are you trying to address? Are you clear about the problem? Therefore, we began writing this chapter by keeping the following questions in mind: *If translational research is the answer, what's the question? Who gets to ask it? How can we better include the key stakeholder constituencies of practitioners and consumers in systems to bridge the gap between research and practice?*

In translational research terminology, our focus in this chapter is on the following questions. See Exhibit 2.1 for definitions of key terms, which are based on Woolf (2008):

- Why are *research-to-practice* models (T1 and T2 translational research) necessary but not sufficient?
- How can T3 (practice-based research, dissemination research, and implementation research) help bridge the research–practice chasm?

EXHIBIT 2.1
What Do We Mean by *Translation* and *Translation Research?*

Translation refers to the process and steps taken to ensure effective and widespread use of evidence-based programs, practices, and policies (Wilson, Brady, & Lesesne, 2011; Wilson & Fridinger, 2008).

Translation research refers to translating research into practice; that is, ensuring that new treatments and research knowledge actually reach the patients or populations for whom they are intended and that they are implemented correctly (Woolf, 2008, p. 211).

- *T1* research is "the transfer of new understandings of disease mechanisms gained in the laboratory into the development of new methods for diagnosis, therapy, and prevention and their first testing in humans" (Woolf, 2008, p. 211).
- *T2* research is "the translation of results from clinical studies into everyday clinical practice and health decision making" (Woolf, 2008, p. 211). T2 research requires different research skills, implementation, and evaluation informed by various areas of public health and social science.
  "T1 struggles more with biological and technological mysteries, trial recruitment, and regulatory concerns. T2 struggles more with human behavior and organizational inertia, infrastructure and resource constraints, and the messiness of proving the effectiveness of 'moving targets' under conditions that investigators cannot fully control" (Woolf, 2008, p. 212).
- T3 research is practice-based research, that is, practice in the field (e.g., in the doctor's office) and dissemination and implementation research (Westfall, Mold, & Fagnan, 2008). According to Woolf (2008), T3 research as described by Westfall is still insufficient because it sees research through the eyes of physicians: "Science informs choices about health habits (e.g., diet, smoking), environmental policy, injury prevention, parenting, healthy workplaces and schools, population health campaigns, and other interventions outside the clinic. The 'practitioners' who apply evidence in these settings include patients, public health administrators, employers, school officials, regulators, product designers, the food industry, and other consumers of evidence" (p. 212).

Woolf proposed that we need "to expand the boundaries of basic science beyond the bench research that T1 typically showcases. Successful health interventions in hospitals, homes, and statehouses require the translation of other basic sciences such as epidemiology, behavioral science, psychology, communication, cognition, social marketing, economics, political science—not only the translation of biotechnological insights and novel therapies. These disciplines deserve their place not only in definitions of basic science but also in funding priorities. Poverty matters as much as proteomics in understanding disease" (p. 212).

- How can the key stakeholder voices of practitioners and consumers be better included in research and practice?

A key strength of health and social science research is the use of rigorous methods to address important questions. A limitation of much research is its lack of its use in practice. Although bodies of research on effective interventions have grown, we have not seen a corresponding increase in the use of effective programs, practices, and policies. Examination of public health and prevention practice in the field suggests that the innovations that have been found most effective in prevention research are not necessarily those most commonly used in practice (e.g., Brownson et al., 2009; Ringwalt et al., 2002; Wandersman & Florin, 2003). To meet the continued health needs of our nation, it would seem prudent to use more of our limited public health resources on what works in prevention and treatment across multiple domains (Rimer, Glanz, & Rasband, 2001).

The issue of designing and promoting evidence-based programs and services is strongly connected to the values and methods used by researchers—who most often value internal validity over external validity and researcher-designed and -driven innovations over community-designed innovations. As such, we think the research questions and approaches and values in wide use have limited utility for practitioners and consumers (i.e., limited external validity). Although we applaud the work of researchers who are attempting to bring research to practice, we think that much is missing if the aim is to improve the health of the American public. For example, researchers who want to bridge research and practice should be concerned with national advocacy organizations (e.g., the American Cancer Society). These organizations survey consumers to assess information needs from groups of different ages, attitudes toward health issues (e.g., obesity) and science, and what practitioners and providers are doing and why. They monitor consumer and practitioner motivations, needs, determinants of action, and responses to social trends (e.g., technology, media, design of community environments to promote physical activity). Researchers often consider organizational advocacy studies to be of lower quality and of limited scientific utility (and certainly there is variability in the quality of these studies). When such studies are done well, however, they provide the kind of information needed to plan for and conduct comprehensive translation efforts precisely because this information can and should inform translation planning, design, and implementation that is feasible and sustainable. Professional organizations and advocacy groups conducting consumer research include the American Academy of Pediatrics (AAP) and the National Campaign to Prevent Teen and Unplanned Pregnancy (National Campaign). AAP conducts periodic surveys of pediatric fellows to better understand the practices of pediatricians across the country with regard to selected topics such as immunization practice. The National Campaign has conducted national representative surveys of parents, teens, and young adults to understand perceptions and beliefs related to teen and unintended pregnancy.

These examples from "consumer or practice" organizations provide a perspective for understanding what information is needed by practitioners at local levels and what is understood and desired by consumers. Although this type of information is not often the subject of study by researchers, it could be useful for informing the development of innovations and of systems to bridge research and practice (as well as the redesign of past innovations that fail to address community needs well). While researchers have adequate methods to address these questions, they often do not ask the necessary questions of certain key stakeholders in their translation efforts.

We begin this chapter by describing research-to-practice models and some limitations. We follow by providing an example of the limitations of research-to-practice models. Then we provide an expansion of the research-to-practice models using a figure to illustrate the need and opportunities for T3 research and beyond from a consumer–practitioner perspective (community-centered/practice-centered). We briefly describe integrating research-to-practice models with community-centered/practice-centered models within the Interactive Systems Framework for Dissemination and Implementation (Wandersman et al., 2008). We conclude with examples of research questions and considerations for the processes needed to establish a consumer–practitioner perspective in translational research. We believe that addressing these questions and considerations will help to bridge the research–practice chasm.

RESEARCH-TO-PRACTICE MODELS

Traditionally, the research–practice gap has been addressed by conceptual models that bring research to practice (Wandersman et al., 2008) and by new approaches that refine research techniques to better support translation of innovations (Glasgow & Emmons, 2007). In their seminal report on prevention research in mental health, the Institute of Medicine (IOM; Mrazek & Haggerty, 1994) developed a five-step model for assessment, intervention, and dissemination: assessing the prevalence and risk and protective factors of a problem area, developing prevention innovations and researching their efficacy and effectiveness, and disseminating these tested innovations into the community (Figure 2.1). This model is a good representation of the dominant paradigm of research to practice. However, the current paradigm has recently been challenged in light of its failure to effectively disseminate at scale. New approaches push researchers to broaden the methods toolbox and more readily embrace external validity as critical to research endeavors. One such tool is the "pragmatic or practical clinical trial" (Glasgow, Magid, Beck, Ritzwoller, & Estabrooks, 2005; Tunis, Stryer, & Clancy, 2003). Advocates of these trials argue that they better approximate reality for consumers, practitioners, and key decision makers by testing multiple alternative clinical innovations using typical participants in typical contexts rather than in unrealistic, tightly controlled contexts. Glasgow et al. (2005) suggested that researchers embrace external validity, while maintaining internal validity, much earlier in the

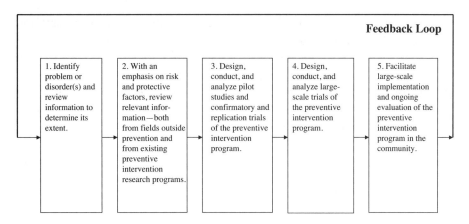

Figure 2.1. Institute of Medicine model of the prevention research cycle. Reprinted from "Bridging the Gap Between Prevention Research and Practice: The Interactive Systems Framework for Dissemination and Implementation," by A. Wandersman, J. Duffy, P. Flaspohler, R. Noonan, K. Lubell, L. Stillman, . . . J. Saul, 2008, *American Journal of Community Psychology, 41,* p. 174. Copyright 2008 by American Psychological Association.

development of trials rather than waiting for effectiveness studies to identify issues. This is because research models strongly emphasize internal validity and often exclude large segments of end users, intended beneficiaries, decision makers, and typical program and service providers by design.

In addition to moving toward future valuable research designs, such as the practical clinical trial, researchers should examine how to promote the translation of existing innovations. Several useful case studies of translation efforts in prevention and public health shed light on this important need (e.g., Brownson et al., 2007; Collins, Phields, & Duncan, 2007; Elliott & Mihalic, 2004; Galbraith et al., 2009; Hawkins et al., 2008) and offer lessons learned as researchers turn their attention toward building environments that support using what works in prevention. (While most of the examples in this chapter are about prevention, we hypothesize that similar issues are generally applicable to clinical services.) Although each of these cases offers unique contributions toward continued efforts that improve prevention practice, most research on interventions contains a pro-innovation bias and may avoid the challenging issues inherent in this bias (Miller & Shinn, 2005). Miller and Shinn (2005) described *pro-innovation bias* as the tendency to overvalue innovations and undervalue indigenous practices and community-developed programs or strategies. In our opinion, this bias combines an emphasis on something new being generated and new programs being initiated by researchers. This bias influences the dominant paradigm on what is acceptable and disseminated by policymakers and funders. When indigenous knowledge, concerns, context, and capacity are undervalued or not considered in translation efforts and innovation trumps community practice, it should be no surprise that the success of translation efforts suffers. To be successful in meeting the translation challenge such that feasible and quality research–based innovations are used by and useful to practitioners and consumers, researchers must expand their worldview and embrace a consumer–practitioner perspective or continue to meet with unsatisfactory progress.

LACK OF UTILIZATION: AN EXAMPLE OF THE LIMITS OF RESEARCH-TO-PRACTICE MODELS

It is widely recognized that obesity is a major public health problem in the United States and that the promotion of physical activity is a major preventive intervention for addressing the problem (e.g., Brownson et al., 2007). In 2001, CDC published *Increasing Physical Activity: A Report on Recommendations of the Task Force on Community Preventive Services* (Community Guide; CDC, 2001). The task force performed a systematic review of 94 physical activity intervention studies published from 1980 to 2000. Based on its review, the task force strongly recommended six interventions (e.g., three behavioral and social approaches: school-based physical education, social support interventions in community settings, and individually adapted health behavior change; see the full review for more details on the inclusion review criteria and methodology).

Given the importance of the problem and the strength of the recommendations, Brownson and colleagues conducted several studies to assess utilization of the Community Guide recommendations for physical activity by state health departments (a major target audience for the guidance). Brownson et al. (2007) surveyed the physical activity contact person in each state and territory (94% response rate). The evidence indicated that of the respondents, 85% had read or seen the guide, 67% had visited the website, 47% had seen printed materials, and 2% had attended training to learn about the guide. In addition, 21% reported that changes in existing programs were made based on the guide and 36% reported that new programs were developed or implemented based on the guide. No detailed information was gathered about the quality of implementation of new programs resulting from the guide. Four characteristics (presence of state funding for physical activity, whether promoting physical activity was a high priority for their health department, presence of adequate staffing, and presence of a supportive state legislature) were statistically associated with use of evidence-based interventions. Notably, three of these factors reflect policies and state government priorities, and the remaining factor relates to staffing capacity for the work.

This suggests that the quality of the evidence base for an innovation is clearly not the only or the dominant factor in adoption.

Later, Brownson and colleagues (Ballew, Brownson, Haire-Joshu, Heath, & Kreuter, 2010) conducted a case study that compared two states with high adoption and implementation of the Community Guide's recommendations for physical activity with two states with low adoption. Key enabling factors for high adoption states included funds and directions from CDC, leadership support, capable staff, and successful partnerships and collaborations. Constraining forces among low adoption states included the Community Guide recommendations for physical activity being too new, participants being too new to current job, lack of time and training in how to use the recommendations, limited funds and other resources, and lack of leadership. Ballew et al. (2010) suggested that a more active approach in promoting the Community Guide recommendations for physical activity would be worthwhile. They described a need for understanding what types of assistance (e.g., more expensive individual contact vs. web-based training) would be useful and where the assistance should be given.

It is clear from Ballew et al. (2010) that the left-to-right approach of research to practice is influenced by policies and organizational factors at the state, community, and individual levels that are complex and perhaps, at times, competing. Many substantial and interacting systems contribute to translation successes and failures. Funding and policies at the macrolevel as well as supports and individual needs (at the meso- and microlevels, respectively) collectively influence the ability and motivation of prevention practitioners to make changes in their everyday work, and hence the feasibility of the intervention in the local context. Although theoretical work such as *Diffusion of Innovations* (Rogers, 2003) provides a useful guide to the factors influencing adoption at these various levels and stages of uptake, the considerations are specific to each type of innovation and utilization context, that is, they are innovation-specific and the factors influencing adoption are complex and systemic, organizational, or individual in nature. We believe the complexity of key influences such as these must be well understood (i.e., well researched) before translation efforts can achieve the desired success. We also believe giving greater emphasis to a consumer–practitioner perspective in these efforts will increase the chances for more rapid positive change at the level of prevention practice because consumers and practitioners can quickly identify the problem areas, develop more feasible solutions, and attend to the interpersonal and attitude-related factors that influence adoption of innovations (Rogers, 2003).

The wisdom gleaned from the Ballew et al. (2010) case study of four health departments is clear and important, and this type of research and the research questions must be furthered. However, it is a post hoc analysis of a passive method of translation in a convenience sample of four health departments. A more proactive effort to identify and address factors related to successful translation should be conducted to inform government (federal and state) efforts to promote the use of the Community Guide recommendations for this and other domains of health. Questions that embrace a consumer–practitioner perspective remain—such as, what do state health department personnel want to know? (They might have questions very different from the questions of those who were surveyed.) Based on the research performed by Ballew et al., state health department personnel might want to know how to get more support from the legislature, political champions, and health department leadership. Limited information is often available regarding what the state health department transmits to local practitioners, to whom they transmit (e.g., local health departments, schools), and what the local practitioner entities need or want to know (or T3 research). What motivates and supports adoption by practitioners? What services do children and families receive, what do they know about alternative services, what motivates them to seek services, and how can the complex needs and motivations of consumers be better incorporated into translational research (expanded T3 research)?

In summary, this example illustrates that extensive intervention research on obesity prevention exists, which public health stakeholders want to see used to its fullest potential. CDC synthesized the research and made a Community Guide available through websites, publications, and conference presentations. However, Ballew et al. (2010) demonstrated that awareness, adoption, and implementation of these recommendations are variable and affected by political factors and organizational and individual capacity. (Note: The Community Guide suggests the importance of administrative structures and local conditions but does not present guidance on what to do about them.) The direction of the CDC work and Ballew's example illustrate a research-to-practice model and some of its advantages and disadvantages. We think that this is a necessary approach but that it is not sufficient to bridge the translational chasm and obtain better public health outcomes.

We believe that a multidirectional framework for bridging research and practice would be helpful. However, multidirectional models challenge how the funding and research communities work. For example, Westfall, Mold, and Fagnan (2007) argued that investigators in the high profile and large NIH Clinical and Translational Science Award grants program (there are 52 programs, many of which receive over $40 million; see http://www.ncrr. nih.gov/clinical_research_resources/clinical_and_translational_science_ awards/interactive_awards_map/awards/) often see the world of practice and the community primarily as a "lab" to do their work and that collaboration is about getting access to people and communities to study the researchers' questions. Although Westfall et al. likely overstated this generalization, the academic community must reflect critically on its approach to innovation and community involvement in the research and translation process. Is the involvement passive? Should the involvement be multidirectional in all phases of applied research so that translation is more successful?

We offer a multidirectional figure using a public health frame as an example of pathways that need development or reinforcement to optimize translation efforts (Figure 2.2). This figure incorporates consumer/practitioner–driven models into a broader representation of translation and translation research. From the left two boxes, NIH and CDC represent funding and research agencies that, similar to other federal agencies (e.g., the U.S. Department of Agriculture), both develop new knowledge and synthesize best practices based on bench and applied science generated from processes described in the IOM model (Mrazek & Haggerty, 1994). Although NIH and CDC differ in their approach to research and application of research findings, it is clear that developing medical or public health scientific innovations (left to right) is necessary but not sufficient. Some have estimated that more than 17 years is necessary for medical innovations to move from paper to practice (Balas & Boren, 2000)—this is unacceptable. The dotted arrows in Figure 2.2 reflect funding or regulatory mandates that typically exist, such as research and applied epidemiology or surveillance funded by CDC and NIH and potential collaborative efforts. Similarly, the products of basic research supported by NIH should be used by CDC and vice versa in attempts to optimize the health of the nation. Using the public health system as an example model, Figure 2.2 represents a basic flow of synthesized research evidence (programs, practices, policies) from CDC or its sister agencies to state health departments for implementation. In some arenas, CDC provides limited funds to state health departments or training to health department staff to utilize the research evidence, but too often there is a passive dissemination that is "automatically" and perhaps "magically" intended to create adoption and active translation of the latest research evidence. The more passive dissemination, if successful, is further transferred to local practitioners within states that may or may not adopt the programs, policies, or practices being encouraged or deliver them with adequate quality. The factors influencing adoption at this level are not well understood, and often the supports needed to understand local complexities and to address them through increasing motivation and skills and developing staff or organizational capacities are not available. The flow of resources and information through the state health department to the practitioner level is too often unidirectional, and rarely are the needs and supports required by practitioners in local communities the subject of inquiry. Thus, the dotted line from practitioners to health departments is desirable but is rarely a formalized, purposeful engagement.

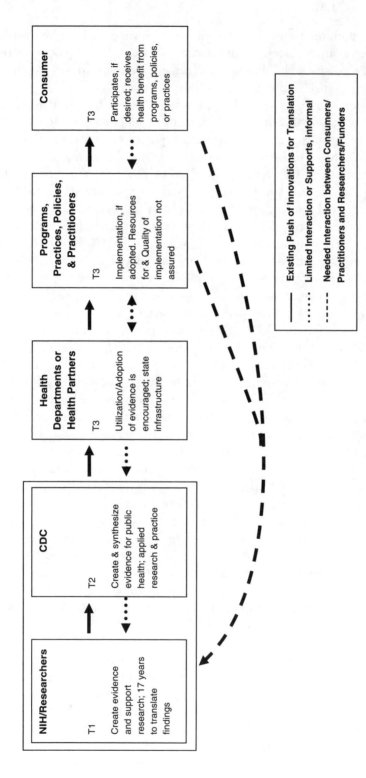

Figure 2.2. Simple visual of translation processes in public health and opportunities to incorporate consumer–practitioner perspectives in translation activities and research.

Last but not least, the consumer of research-based innovations is most often perceived as a passive recipient. However, consumers are not passive; in fact, they are very active. The dotted line from consumers to practitioners is also rarely formalized or attended to despite the ultimate need for consumers to "consume" the innovations. In a similar vein, funders and researchers on the left side of the figure are several layers removed from consumers and practitioners, although bridging the distance would be useful. Funders and researchers must challenge themselves to value these groups, to work for them and with them—not at them—and to do this routinely with an eye for developing research evidence that consumers want; that practitioners can buy into, support, and implement; and that consumers and practitioners are motivated to use because it efficiently meets important needs in their local community. The dashed lines from consumers and practitioners to NIH and CDC and the researchers they fund represent a need to embrace a consumer–practitioner perspective in solving the problem of bridging research and practice.

INTEGRATING RESEARCH-TO-PRACTICE MODELS AND COMMUNITY-CENTERED MODELS: THE INTERACTIVE SYSTEMS FRAMEWORK FOR DISSEMINATION AND IMPLEMENTATION

Effectively bridging research and practice is a difficult process that has inspired much research as well as several models and frameworks (e.g., Fixsen, Naoom, Blase, Friedman, & Wallace, 2005; Greenhalgh, Robert, Macfarlane, Bate, & Kyriakidou, 2004; Wandersman et al., 2008). These models and others are informed by research findings but often lack a strong empirical basis of their own. In many cases they rely heavily on reflection on experience or documentation of case studies offered by researchers who critically examine lessons learned from efforts in the field. The Interactive Systems Framework for Dissemination and Implementation (ISF; Wandersman et al., 2008) is one such model. In developing the ISF, Wandersman et al. (2008) examined research-to-practice models and community-centered models. *Research-to-practice models* begin with the researchers and research; *community-centered models* begin with the world of practice. The dominant models in understanding the relationship between research and practice are those starting with research, such as the IOM model of the prevention research cycle (Figure 2.1). In contrast, community-centered models "begin with the community and ask what it needs in terms of scientific information and capacity-building to produce effective interventions" (Wandersman, 2003, p. 230). The models suggest that understanding capacity, as well as capacity in context, is central in addressing the gap between research and practice (Flaspohler, Duffy,

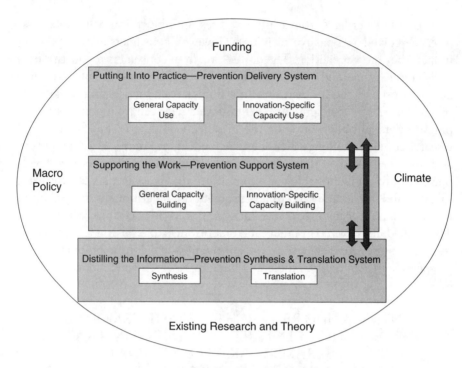

Figure 2.3. The Interactive Systems Framework for Dissemination and Implementation. Reprinted from "Bridging the Gap Between Prevention Research and Practice: The Interactive Systems Framework for Dissemination and Implementation," by A. Wandersman, J. Duffy, P. Flaspohler, R. Noonan, K. Lubell, L. Stillman, . . . J. Saul, 2008, *American Journal of Community Psychology, 41,* p. 174. Copyright 2008 by American Psychological Association.

Wandersman, Stillman, & Maras, 2008; Goodman et al., 1998; Miller & Shinn, 2005; Wandersman, 2003). Two types of capacity (defined here as *skills* and *motivation*) are necessary at the individual, organizational, and community levels: (a) the capacity required to deliver a specific innovation and (b) the capacity for effective structure and functioning that promotes innovation and keeps the individuals, organizations, and communities viable (e.g., Livet & Wandersman, 2005). Thus, capacity issues are complex as they interact within and across levels and evolve over time.

The ISF (shown in Figure 2.3) is intended to illuminate the arrow between boxes four and five in the IOM model of the research-to-practice cycle (shown in Figure 2.1) by detailing the systems and functions that should work bidirectionally to bridge science and practice. The ISF consists of three systems: the Prevention Synthesis and Translation System, the Prevention Support System, and the Prevention Delivery System. The term *system* is used broadly here to describe a set of activities and actors that may vary in the degree to which they are systematic or coherently organized. The function of the Prevention Synthesis and Translation System is conceptualized as distilling information about innovations and preparing them for implementation by end users. The information can be derived from efficacy and effectiveness studies, health services research, or community-based participatory research. The function of the Prevention Support System is conceptualized as supporting the work of those who will put the innovations into practice. Successful translation requires a variety of supporting systems, structures, and processes (e.g., training and technical assistance) that support general capacity or innovation-specific capacity. The primary function of the Prevention Delivery System is the implementation of innovations (e.g., delivery of programs) in the field. It is important to note that the "delivery system" is not just a venue for delivery but also encompasses consumers and practitioners who wield their own attitudes, motivations, knowledge, and skills that influence the decision to adopt innovations and affect actual implementation. In summary, the ISF is centered on the infrastructure and interaction of systems and stakeholders (e.g., prevention practitioners, organizations that provide support to practitioners, funders, and researchers and evaluators) needed to carry out the functions necessary for dissemination and implementation to take place. Examples of the ISF in action are reported in the 2008 special issue of the *American Journal of Community Psychology* (Vol. 41, Nos. 3–4) dedicated to the ISF and coedited by Wandersman, Flaspohler, and Saul.

The ISF was designed to accommodate multiple perspectives (e.g., the perspectives of the funder, researcher, practitioner, and technical assistance provider) and the need to consider them in an interactive, bidirectional fashion. The ISF also highlights the importance of capacity (both general and innovation-specific) within the various systems involved in the dissemination and implementation of innovations in new settings. It draws explicitly on the knowledge and expertise of prevention practitioners, funding agencies, support agencies, and researchers from the fields of prevention and dissemination. This combination of perspectives has yielded a framework that we believe is useful for people in each role. The ISF includes the activities or functions carried out by people in multiple types of roles. Although individuals working within any or all of the three systems can identify their own work, they also can see how their work relates to work done throughout the system. The ISF also highlights the need for bidirectional communication among the different stakeholders in the system, such as funders, practitioners, trainers, and researchers. An upcoming special issue of the *American Journal of Community Psychology* on the ISF (Wandersman, Flaspohler, Lesesne, Puddy, & Smith, 2011) will include case examples in which consumers are taken into greater account in the translation process.

The ISF can guide thinking on how to shift the balance in current research-to-practice directions toward more multidirectional, researcher–consumer/practitioner perspectives. Translational research can provide data on how to make research innovations meet needs and fit communities well so that innovations are feasible locally. Starting from the Prevention Delivery System, researchers could work their way down the ISF using the research methods to better understand the needs, motivations, and context in which delivery of innovations might occur. Findings should influence the development of innovations, as well as the retrofitting of older innovations that did not adequately take into account the complex context of local implementation, to make interventions more effective and more likely to be adopted and sustained because they meet local needs and capacities. Below we offer some ideas for future research that are guided by the ISF and represent a value for consumers and practitioners.

We propose that there be much more intensive study of what practitioners, consumers, and communities need, want, understand, and can use in prevention practice. Absent a clear understanding of the main settings in which prevention programming is delivered; the types of programs, practices, and policies being used across settings; and the interest and willingness of practitioners to learn about or adopt science-based programs, it will be difficult to systematically influence the widespread adoption and quality implementation of innovations as "pushed" from research onto practice. Drawing on our earlier public health framework, we provide examples of translational research questions guided by the ISF. We note that (a) these questions should be customized for different health and human services domains (e.g., important facets of obesity prevention, teen pregnancy prevention, and immunization may differ and require variations on the question) and (b) the answers may be different in different domains. In brief, developing a comprehensive approach to translational research will require ideographic (unique) and nomothetic (common) questions and answers across domains.

Prevention Delivery System (Practitioners and Consumers)

- What are the needs, perceptions, motivations, and reinforcements for practitioners in adopting innovations and for consumers in engaging in active use of innovations?
- Who are the key delivery system stakeholders (e.g., the practitioners and consumers relevant to a given program, policy, or practice innovation if it were to be adopted)?

- What are the characteristics of delivery systems and how would innovations be perceived in these contexts? Which systems are "open" to adopting innovations? Under what circumstances would system stakeholders be motivated to change their programs, policies, or practice?

Prevention Support System (Capacity Building and Infrastructure Supports)

- What types of training for practitioners and consumers are needed to support innovations? Which supports predict capacity building success, capacity use, and quality implementation of programs, policies, and practice innovations?
- What maintenance supports are needed once high-level general and innovation-specific capacities are achieved?

Prevention Synthesis and Translation System (Active Creation and Dissemination of Practitioner/Consumer-Friendly Innovations)

- How can we more effectively disseminate these resources to ensure that important audiences learn about what the research is telling us? What do practitioners and consumers need to know about an innovation to use it locally?
- What opportunities exist to retrofit an innovation for more successful translation? How can we optimize the chance for adoption of evidence-based programs, policies, and practices by adapting them to better fit needs of practitioners and consumers?

CONCLUSION

To fully engage in translation research in answering these and other questions, important dimensions and processes for embracing a consumer–practitioner perspective will need to be considered. Exhibit 2.2 offers a preliminary look at the factors that can help or hinder use of this perspective as well as the processes and potential benefits of taking a consumer–practitioner perspective into translation work. Shifting our perspective will not be easy, but funders, researchers, and translation partners can consider the processes we describe in Exhibit 2.2 to begin this journey. We believe that translation activities and research (expanded T3 in particular) that embrace consumers and practitioners fully will optimize the chances for successful translation at local levels. They will also illuminate the needs to be addressed in the three systems of the ISF that undergird translation action. It is not our methods

EXHIBIT 2.2
Dimensions of a Consumer–Practitioner Perspective: Barriers, Facilitators, Processes, and Effects

Factors that deter consumer–practitioner perspective

- Consumers and practitioners may or may not perceive "issue" as a priority problem to be addressed; policymakers and funders may or may not perceive "issue" as important.
- Consumers and practitioners encompass a mass of diverse stakeholders to engage; the scale and diverse, horizontal lines of authority make engagement difficult.
- The time, cost, and difficulty of engaging consumers and practitioners may be prohibitive and are often not supported by federal and state funders.

Factors that promote consumer–practitioner perspective

- Consumers and practitioners are the beneficiaries and necessary actors for quality improvement and translation action.
- Consumers and practitioners have motivations, needs, and perspectives that can help or hinder success in quality improvement and translation action.
- Consumers and practitioners are the key partners in almost all translation actions (and they can support policy and priorities in their community leadership).

Processes that engage consumers and practitioners

- Consumers and practitioners are the research priority population—exploratory surveys, interviews, town halls, and focus groups should start all translation efforts. Genuine concern for the motivations, resources, risks and benefits, training needs, and organizational limitations must be present *before initiating development of innovations or attempting to transfer innovations into communities.*
- Implementation research, documentation, and capacity building needs must be developed, tested, and vetted by consumers and practitioners and relevant leadership. Efforts should involve a diversity of the key consumer and practitioner stakeholders engaged early in the process.
- Consumers and practitioners are the key partners in almost all translation actions (and they can support policy and priorities in their community leadership); thus, they must be treated with equal respect and given nontrivial authority over their own actions and priorities.

Potential effects of consumer–practitioner engagement

- Diverse consumer and practitioner stakeholders are well understood in relation to the innovation; for example, using *Getting to Outcomes* steps (Wandersman, Imm, Chinman, & Kaftarian, 2000), we have a picture of the needs, goals, practices, fit, capacity, plan, implementation, evaluation, and sustainability of consumers and practitioners in their own communities, in their own words.
- Funders, leaders, and other stakeholders can target limited resources on improving quality and translation efforts toward issues that are important to communities and in contexts capable of adopting innovations.
- Translation efforts can be designed to optimize consumer and practitioner motivation, resources, capacity building and training needs, implementation supports, and organizational needs *prior to initiating innovations or attempting to retrofit and transfer innovations into communities.*
- Create a network of consumers and practitioners that are boundary spanners, partners with researchers so that future innovations are sensitive *by design* to the needs and contexts of eventual adoption and longer-term sustainability. This respects consumers and practitioners as more than just "participants"—they are partners in solving community problems using science as a tool to meet their own needs.

of inquiry that need the most attention, it is the critical reflection on who gets to ask what questions. We propose that the consumer–practitioner perspective is an extremely important lens through which research should view translation efforts and guide the development of innovations. If we further develop this lens, we are more likely to ask the right questions and embrace the complex needs and motivations of consumers and practitioners as they work to solve local problems. In line with the ISF, funders and researchers should help build the capacities of practitioners and consumers to participate actively in developing the translational research questions that are answered and in accessing and using the evidence base to achieve outcomes more effectively and efficiently.

REFERENCES

Balas, E. A., & Boren, S. A. (2000). Managing clinical knowledge for health care improvement. In Bemmel, J., & A. T. McCray (Eds.), *Yearbook of medical informatics 2000: Patient-centered systems* (pp. 65–70). Stuttgart, Germany: Schattauer Verlagsgesellschaft.

Ballew, P., Brownson, R. C., Haire-Joshu, D., Heath, G. W., & Kreuter, M. W. (2010). Dissemination of effective physical activity interventions: Are we applying the evidence? *Health Education Research, 25,* 185–198. doi:10.1093/her/cyq003

Brownson, R. C., Ballew, P., Brown, K., Elliott, M., Haire-Joshu, D., Heath, G., & Kreuter, M. (2007). The effect of disseminating evidence-based interventions that promote physical activity to health departments. *American Journal of Public Health, 97,* 1900–1907. doi:10.2105/AJPH.2006.090399

Brownson, R. C., Fielding, J. E., & Maylan, C. M. (2009). Evidence-based public health: A fundamental concept for public health practice. *Annual Review of Public Health, 30,* 175–201. doi:10.1146/annurev.publhealth.031308.100134

Centers for Disease Control and Prevention. (2001). *Increasing physical activity. A report on recommendations of the Task Force on Community Preventive Services.* Retrieved from http://www.cdc.gov/mmwr/preview/mmwrhtml/rr5018a1.htm

Collins, C., Phields, M. E., & Duncan, T. (2007). An agency capacity model to facilitate implementation of evidence-based behavioral interventions by community-based organizations. *Journal of Public Health Management and Practice, 13*(Suppl.), S16–S23.

Elliott, D. S., & Mihalic, S. (2004). Issues in disseminating and replicating effective prevention programs. *Prevention Science, 5*(1), 47–53. doi:10.1023/B:PREV.0000013981.28071.52

Fixsen, D. L., Naoom, S. F., Blase, K. A., Friedman, R. M., & Wallace, F. (2005). *Implementation research: A synthesis of the literature.* Tampa, FL: University of South Florida, Louis de la Parte Florida Mental Health Institute, The National Implementation Research Network.

Flaspohler, P., Duffy, J., Wandersman, A., Stillman, L., & Maras, M. A. (2008). Unpacking prevention capacity: An intersection of research-to-practice models and community-centered models. *American Journal of Community Psychology, 41*(3–4), 182–196. doi:10.1007/s10464-008-9162-3

Galbraith, J. S., Stanton, B., Boekeloo, B., King, W., Desmond, S., Howard, D., . . . Carey, J. W. (2009). Exploring implementation and fidelity of evidence-based behavioral interventions for HIV prevention: Lessons learned from the Focus on Kids diffusion case study. *Health Education & Behavior, 36,* 532–549. doi:10.1177/1090198108315366

Glasgow, R. E., & Emmons, K. M. (2007). How can we increase translation of research into practice? Types of evidence needed. *Annual Review of Public Health, 28,* 413–433. doi:10.1146/annurev.publhealth.28.021406.144145

Glasgow, R. E., Magid, D. J., Beck, A., Ritzwoller, D., & Estabrooks, P. A. (2005). Practical clinical trials for translating research to practice: Design and measurement recommendations. *Medical Care, 43,* 551–557. doi:10.1097/01.mlr.0000163645.41407.09

Goodman, R. M., Speers, M., McLeroy, K., Fawcett, S., Kegler, M., Parker, E., . . . Wallerstein, N. (1998). Identifying and defining the dimensions of community capacity to provide a basis for measurement. *Health Education & Behavior, 25,* 258–278. doi:10.1177/109019819802500303

Greenhalgh, T., Robert, G., Macfarlane, F., Bate, P., & Kyriakidou, O. (2004). Diffusion of innovations in service organizations: Systematic review and recommendations. *Milbank Quarterly, 82,* 581–629. doi:10.1111/j.0887-378X.2004.00325.x

Hawkins, J. D., Catalano, R. F., Arthur, M. W., Egan, E., Brown, E. C., Abbott, R. D., & Murray, D. M. (2008). Testing Communities That Care: The rationale, design, and behavioral baseline equivalences of the Community Youth Development Study. *Prevention Science, 9,* 178–190. doi:10.1007/s11121-008-0092-y

Livet, M., & Wandersman, A. (2005). Organizational functioning: Facilitating effective interventions and increasing the odds of programming success. In D. M. Fetterman & A. Wandersman (Eds.), *Empowerment evaluation principles in practice* (pp. 123–154). New York, NY: Guilford Press.

Miller, R. L., & Shinn, M. (2005). Learning from communities: Overcoming difficulties in dissemination of prevention and promotion efforts. *American Journal of Community Psychology, 35*(3–4), 169–183. doi:10.1007/s10464-005-3395-1

Mrazek, P., & Haggerty, R. (1994). *Reducing risks for mental disorders: Frontiers for preventive intervention research.* Washington, DC: National Academy Press.

Rimer, B. K., Glanz, K., & Rasband, G. (2001). Searching for evidence about health education and health behavior interventions. *Health Education & Behavior, 28,* 231–248. doi:10.1177/109019810102800208

Ringwalt, C. L., Ennet, S., Vincus, A., Thorne, J., Rohrbach, L. A., & Simons-Rudolph, A. (2002). The prevalence of effective substance use prevention curricula in U.S. middle schools. *Prevention Science, 3,* 257–265. doi:10.1023/A:1020872424136

Rogers, E. M. (2003). *Diffusion of innovations* (5th ed.). New York, NY: Free Press.

Tunis, S. R., Stryer, D. B., & Clancy, C. M. (2003). Practical clinical trials: increasing the value of clinical research for decision making in clinical and health policy. JAMA, *290*, 1624–1632. doi:10.1001/jama.290.12.1624

Wandersman, A. (2003). Community science: Bridging the gap between science and practice with community-centered models. *American Journal of Community Psychology, 31*, 227–242. doi:10.1023/A:1023954503247

Wandersman, A., Duffy, J., Flaspohler, P., Noonan, R., Lubell, K., Stillman, L., . . . Saul, J. (2008). Bridging the gap between prevention research and practice: The Interactive Systems Framework for Dissemination and Implementation. *American Journal of Community Psychology, 41*, 171–181. doi:10.1007/s10464-008-9174-z

Wandersman, A., Flaspohler, P., Lesesne, C., Puddy, R., & Smith, E. (2011). *Advancing the Interactive Systems Framework for dissemination and implementation.* Manuscript submitted for publication.

Wandersman, A., & Florin, P. (2003). Community interventions and effective prevention. *American Psychologist, 58*, 441–448. doi:10.1037/0003-066X.58.6-7.441

Wandersman, A., Imm, P., Chinman, M., & Kaftarian, S. (2000). Getting to outcomes: A results-based approach to accountability. *Evaluation and Program Planning, 23*, 389–395. doi:10.1016/S0149-7189(00)00028-8

Westfall, J. M., Mold, J., & Fagnan, L. (2007). Practice-based research—"Blue highways" on the NIH roadmap. JAMA, *297*, 403–406. doi:10.1001/jama.297.4.403

Wilson, K. M., Brady, T. J., & Lesesne, C. A. (2011). An organizing framework for translation in public health: CDC's National Center for Chronic Disease Prevention and Health Promotion's knowledge to action framework. *Preventing Chronic Disease, 8*(2), 1–7.

Wilson, K. M., & Fridinger, F. (2008). Focusing on public health: A different look at translating research to practice. *Journal of Women's Health, 17*, 173–179. doi:10.1089/jwh.2007.0699

Woolf, S. H. (2008). The meaning of translational research and why it matters. JAMA, *299*, 211–213. doi:10.1001/jama.2007.26

3

OPPORTUNITIES FOR AND CHALLENGES OF TRANSLATING EDUCATIONAL AND DEVELOPMENTAL RESEARCH INTO POLICY AND INTERVENTION

ROBERT CROSNOE

Translational research connotes different things to different audiences. In the medical sciences, it generally refers to some form of the "bench to bed-side enterprise" (Woolf, 2008, p. 211). In the social and behavioral sciences, it primarily concerns efforts to "bridge the gap between empirical research on human problems and practical programs to address them" (Sabir et al., 2006, p. 833). Regardless of the conceptualization, translational research represents a somewhat uneasy relationship among professional fields with different approaches to and stakes in public health, education, and other societal institutions and population patterns (Huston, 2008). As explained by Sabir et al. (2006), the uneasiness of this relationship is rooted in many fairly mundane practical issues. On the one hand, practitioners and policymakers lack the time or the training to incorporate research into their intervention strategies and might believe that research, especially national-level research, lacks relevance to what they do on a daily basis. On the other hand, social and

The research discussed in this chapter was supported by the Foundation for Child Development young scholars fellowships, the William T. Grant Foundation, and the National Institute of Child Health and Human Development (R01 HD055359, PI: Robert Crosnoe; R03 HD047378-01, PI: Robert Crosnoe; R24 HD042849, PI: Mark Hayward).

behavioral scientists often perceive, accurately or not, that applied work will not be as highly valued by their colleagues as their pursuits of "pure" science and fear that it will not produce the tangible markers of professional success (e.g., peer-reviewed publications) that they need to get ahead in their careers. Indeed, these concerns may be great enough that we are experiencing something of a "brain drain" in translational research, losing capable social and behavioral scientists with something to offer to the research–policy nexus.

My own career has been something of a microcosm of these inherent difficulties in the field of translational research. Motivated to get a PhD in sociology by an abiding interest in social justice and a (perhaps naïve) belief in the power of public policy to do good, I entered a graduate program that offered no training in applied work or policy analysis and, indeed, implicitly devalued such pursuits. From there, I set out on a traditional tenure-oriented professional track with the usual pressures and time constraints that limited my ability to branch out from basic theory-driven, policy-agnostic research. By the time that I was exposed to professional groups and networks that encouraged me to return to my original aim of being a translational researcher, I realized that I simply did not know how to do it; specifically, how to connect to and work with policymakers and practitioners in effective ways. An added challenge was the crosscurrents occurring in my major fields of study. Sociologists and psychologists had begun to at least talk more about the need for translational research. At the same time, educational science was undergoing some growing pains regarding the nature of educational research and its role in informing policy, including a push at the federal level to make educational research—long a major domain of translation—more basic and "scientific" (Shavelson & Towne, 2006). Thus, years after leaving my formal training as a researcher, I had to undergo a whole new learning process, an ambiguous and unstructured one that eventually led me to change my expectations of and goals for translational research.

The developmentally oriented research that I have conducted on education and educational inequality in the United States over the past decade offers a window into this learning process. Disparities in the educational system related to family socioeconomic circumstances, race and ethnicity, and immigration represent an important and timely policy issue. My own empirical studies of this issue, initially as a basic researcher, proved to be the venue in which I began to better understand the two-way connection between research and policy and, eventually, figure out and work my way through some of the basic problems that undermine this connection. In this chapter, I give an overview of pressing educational challenges, describe what I have done about these challenges in terms of basic research, explain how I have started to take steps to translate this research, and detail the lessons I have learned along the way.

EDUCATION AND EDUCATIONAL INEQUALITY

In *The State of Americans*, Urie Bronfenbrenner and his colleagues wrote, "There is no more critical indicator of the future of society than the character, competence, and integrity of its youth" (Bronfenbrenner, McClelland, Wethington, Moen, & Ceci, 1996, p. 1). This general sentiment is crystallized in the specific case of the American educational system, which was designed to give individual youths the chance to get ahead in life and, in the aggregate, to promote the economic and social interests of the United States. How young people fare in the system, therefore, helps to determine how the nation fares, which shapes the futures of young people and so on (Arum, 2000; Schneider, 2007). Today, several population-level trends have converged to alter the link between education and socioeconomic attainment in ways that create a major paradox in this culturally valued role of education in the individual life course and society at large. In short, the personal and social benefits of educational attainment are increasing, but so too are the obstacles to attaining an education.

Supply, Demand, and Returns in Contemporary Education

Over the past several decades, the American economy has been transformed by sweeping macrolevel economic forces (Fischer & Hout, 2006; Goldin & Katz, 2008). Specifically, the economy has shifted from an industrial phase driven by heavy manufacturing to a postindustrial phase rooted in the service and information sectors. In the resulting labor market, white collar jobs with benefits and wage growth have increased in number, as have unstable, insecure jobs with no clear trajectory of advancement. The options between these high and low ends (e.g., "good" blue collar jobs, such as in manufacturing) have narrowed considerably, making social mobility that much more difficult for young people in the low and middle portions of the socioeconomic gradient (Bernhardt, Morris, Handcock, & Scott, 2001; Lemieux, 2006; Massey, 1996). This economic change has driven other population trends—including growing income inequality, greater instability in normative job sequences, and stagnant and declining real wages—and has been exacerbated by cyclical economic dynamics that created the 2009–2010 recession (Bernhardt et al., 2001; Goldin & Katz, 2008; Lemieux, 2006).

All of this change has altered the school-to-work sequence in contemporary cohorts of American youth. In short, according to Fischer and Hout (2006), higher education has become the dividing line of society. In the past, a high school diploma was sufficient for entry into the manufacturing sector, which, because of unionization, benefits, wage growth, and security, promoted socioeconomic stability and social mobility. Now, the reduction of the manufacturing sector and the growth of the information technology sector have greatly increased demand for specific skills and credentials, leading to a rise in returns to higher education. Indeed, the economic benefits of a post–high school degree are now at an all-time high (Diprete & Buchmann, 2006; Goldin & Katz, 2008; Heckman, Lochner, & Todd, 2007; Lemieux, 2006).

Importantly, such returns vary across different sectors and levels of higher education, with returns to advanced degrees growing more rapidly than returns to baccalaureate degrees, and similar trends related to the selectivity of universities and to math, science, business, and technology over other fields of study (Goldin & Katz, 2008; Hoxby, 2004; Schneider, 2007). The rising demand among employers for workers with higher educations should lead to an increase in supply in the form of growing rates of college matriculation. Yet, increased supply has primarily occurred in the upper tail of the socioeconomic distribution. In other words, youth from more advantaged family backgrounds have posted the most significant increases in college matriculation and graduation. Moreover, whatever increased supply that has occurred has not been as big as it should have been given the increased demand for higher education in the labor market (Goldin & Katz, 2008; Kane, 2007). This unexpected supply–demand dynamic is rooted in the increasing tuition costs of higher education, a decrease in public funding and education assistance, wage stagnation, and a failure of the quantity of university and college slots to keep up with population growth in young American cohorts (Fischer & Hout, 2006; Kane, 2007; Turner & Bound, 2006). Thus, the cohort of youth graduating from high school now faces greater need for higher education and greater constraints against entering higher education, a situation that is driving larger patterns of inequality in the population.

Role of Educational Research

This contemporary educational challenge poses problems on individual, community, and population levels, and, as such, motivates clear policy goals—raising the overall flow of young people into higher education while also reducing socioeconomic and related disparities in this flow. These goals have, in turn, sparked a good deal of social and behavioral research on the pre-K through 12th grade educational system and, more generally, on the early life course. This research takes several different forms. Some of this research has no clear policy agenda, although it is certainly policy relevant. For example, the qualitative work of sociologist Annette Lareau (2004) advances theoretical understanding of how cultural differences across social groups engender parenting differences that provide some young people with competitive advantages over their peers in school. Other portions of this body of research are more explicitly aimed at informing policy and practice. The various studies by economists and other researchers compiled in the 2004 volume *College Choices* (Hoxby, 2004) provide a good collective example. Finally, still others are deeply tied to programmatic efforts, as exemplified by program evaluations and research-based educational interventions (Gandara, 2002; Raver et al., 2008). All of this research has highlighted crucial social and institutional issues in the path to college (and inequalities along this path). Next, I touch on four of these issues as a way of discussing the link between research and policy.

First, a growing consensus in economics, neuroscience, and psychology holds that early childhood is a foundational period for the development of skills that carry youth into adulthood (Knudsen, Heckman, Cameron, & Shonkoff, 2006). This consensus is, in part, grounded in long-standing, well-documented, and consistent patterns that have emerged from cross-disciplinary empirical observation. The patterns suggest that the cumulative nature of instruction, course placement, expectations, and learning can cause the differences in children's school readiness and their academic progress in the early years of elementary school to compound into large disparities in end-of-school outcomes (Alexander, Entwisle, & Olson, 2007; Pianta, Cox, & Snow, 2007). This theoretically grounded research base, in turn, has fueled early interventions as well as economic arguments about the heightened returns of early investment (Heckman, 2006; Karloy, Kilburn, & Cannon, 2006; Ludwig & Sawhill, 2007). In addition to Head Start and Early Head Start, the universal pre-K programs being enacted in numerous states, efforts to align pre-K and elementary school curricula and standards, and the formulation of state and federal school readiness goals represent products of and motivation for basic and applied research, including the research coming out of the new Early Childhood Longitudinal Studies from the National Center for Education Statistics (Crosnoe, 2006; Fuller, 2007; Gormley, Gayer, Phillips, & Dawson, 2005; Love et al., 2005).

Second, family–school relations represent one way that research on family processes can be linked to educational policy action. Although parenting is clearly of major importance in the education of young people, it is difficult to manipulate externally on the larger scale (e.g., policies targeting parenting behavior) because of practical, ethical, and political expedience issues (Crosnoe, 2011; Huston, 2008). Aspects of parenting that connect to the mission of schools, and therefore can be facilitated by schools, offer a way around this problem. Not surprisingly, then, these parenting behaviors—such as parents' support of learning at home and involvement in school activities (e.g., PTA, teacher meetings)—have long been studied by social and behavioral scientists and are perhaps the most commonly examined aspects of parenting among educational researchers (Cheadle, 2008; Hill & Tyson, 2009). At the same time, such aspects of family–school relations are also among the most commonly targeted family and parenting factors in educational policy, albeit with mixed success, culminating in the parental involvement (or family–school compact) provision of No Child Left Behind (Domina, 2005; Epstein, 2005). Again, what is important is the two-way exchange between research and policy, with theories of family–school relations producing empirical evidence that influences policy and program implementation that, in turn, shapes theoretical understanding and empirical examination of family–school relations.

Third, although family dynamics and other aspects of interpersonal relations are commonly studied by social and behavioral scientists, they are much less often studied by educational researchers with an explicit goal of informing educational policy (Dornbusch, Glasgow, & Lin, 1996). The latter group tends to focus on the structural and organizational aspects of social institutions and contexts that historically have been more subject to policy intervention (Chubb & Moe, 1990; Clotfelter, Ladd, & Vigdor, 2007). As one example, school size is an issue that connects with theoretical interests of researchers in social integration, belongingness, and alienation as well as with policy considerations about economies of scale, the curriculum, and extracurricular activities. As such, school size has been the focus of a good deal of give and take between researchers and policymakers over the years, from support of school consolidation to smaller schools and schools within schools (Barker & Gump, 1964; Lee & Ready, 2007). As another example, growing concerns about the competitiveness of American students in the global marketplace have led to calls for school reform, which, in turn, have generated empirical research supporting specific kinds of school reorganization and curricular redesign (Attewell & Domina, 2008; National Commission on Excellence in Education, 1983). High schools look different today than they did 2 decades ago, and this is due in part to the new knowledge base, arising from the social and behavioral sciences, about what helps and hurts young people on the path to college.

Fourth, the transition between high school and college has proved to be one of the most powerful meeting points for research and policy in education (Tierney et al., 2009). For the most part, research has focused on the obstacles that students—especially those from historically disadvantaged groups—face in navigating high school curricula to get to (and be prepared for) college and, moreover, the social or institutional resources that help them overcome these obstacles (Morgan, 2005; Sadler & Tai, 2007; Schneider, 2007). Much of this empirical research is grounded in the social, cultural, and human capital theoretical traditions. These theoretical underpinnings are also reflected in many of the large-scale interventions that target "leakage" points in the pipeline to college and that emphasize social support and access to information networks of social ties as key to keeping young people, especially poor minority youth, on track for college matriculation and completion. For example, High School Puente, a school-based program in California that aims to increase the college-going of Latina and Latino adolescents, is predicated on the culturally sensitive mentoring and guidance of adults with inside knowledge of the educational system (Gandara, 2002). National programs, such as Upward Bound or Gear Up, follow a similar socially focused model of intervention (Swail & Perna, 2002; Tierney et al., 2009).

Despite the cross-pollination of research and policy around these four educational issues, active partnerships between research and policy/practice are still the exception rather than the rule. In general, such cross-pollination does not broadly occur in a systematic way, and it is not often taught formally in graduate programs outside of schools of public policy, social work, and education. Large-scale policies that are not sufficiently based on scientific evidence and research enterprises that are not sufficiently cognizant of the challenges faced by stakeholders in enacting policies and programs are more likely to occur. A good example is No Child Left Behind, the sweeping federal legislation on educational reform, which did not incorporate many scientific voices in its development but generated much scientific criticism after the fact (Epstein, 2005). Thus, regarding the pipeline to college, translational research has made a great deal of progress but has a long way to go. At least some of the burden must be carried by the researchers trying to do the translating and not just the stakeholders who are the intended target of that translation.

ATTEMPTS AT TRANSLATION

Since leaving graduate school a decade ago, I have been actively involved as a researcher in the field of education and educational inequality in general and in the subfields surrounding the four specific issues just described. By researcher, I mean primarily as a basic researcher—one who draws on theory to organize empirical analyses with the ultimate goal of producing knowledge—rather than as a translational researcher. More recently this has changed as I see myself moving, at least in spirit, toward a translational research model. This evolution is likely something that many of today's graduate students and early career scholars in psychology, sociology, and related fields will undergo in the coming years, and so my experience may be instructive for them.

Developing a Research Program

Starting out, I focused on adolescence and high school, with a strictly quantitative, national-level approach that integrated my training in sociology of education, social demography, and developmental psychology. I only paid peripheral attention to the policy implications of my work. What fascinated me was how the formal processes of education (e.g., instruction, curriculum, academic progress) so crucial to socioeconomic attainment were linked in positive and negative ways to the more informal processes (e.g., social relations) of high school life. The research program that I built over the years applied the life course framework in examining the connection between the educational pathways of young people, their general socioemotional development, and health, and how this connection contributed to socioeconomic and racial and ethnic (including immigration-related) disparities in educational attainment (Crosnoe, 2001). I focused primarily on peer relations and their role, through adolescent identity development, in disrupting and supporting adolescents' academic progress within and across demographic groups (Crosnoe, 2004). Eventually, I came to see that the adolescent–high school phenomena that I was studying could be better understood by looking at how students evolved over time and, consequently, I slowly shifted my focus to childhood and, in particular, the transition into elementary school (Crosnoe, 2006).

The most frequent criticism I received about this work was that it was theoretically important but practically useless. Understanding peer dynamics, the criticism went, was an important part of elucidating the social stratification of developmental and educational trajectories, but it did not offer concrete guidance about what schools or communities could do to improve educational performance rates or to reduce educational disparities. I have come to think of this as the policy dilemma of developmentally oriented educational and health research. As a result, I did not, for many years, consider translation to be a "doable" goal for me in my career despite my belief that such translation was a major value of social and behavioral research.

A turning point for me was that the research that I was doing selected me into professional networks that explicitly encouraged and supported efforts to craft basic research in a policy-oriented way. Such groups included the William T. Grant Foundation Scholars program, the Foundation for Child Development Changing Faces of America's Youth early career program, and the Eunice Kennedy Shriver National Institute of Child Health and Human Development (NICHD) Early Child Care Research Network. The message that I received in these groups was not that I should turn away from the research questions that interested me simply because they did not appear to be policy relevant. Instead, it was that I needed to figure out how to answer those questions in ways that highlighted their policy relevance. The research that I conducted as part of my W. T. Grant project under the guidance of two established translational researchers—the developmental psychologist Aletha Huston and the sociologist of education Barbara Schneider—is perhaps the best example of how I slowly worked through the issues faced by many young scholars who are interested in policy but have no training in how to pursue that interest.

Changing Directions

The purpose of this W. T. Grant project was to understand how socio-economic disparities in the math and science curricula in secondary school, major conduits of college-going, were related to differences in the social support that socioeconomically advantaged and disadvantaged youth drew from their relationships with peers, parents, and other adults. On a basic level, this project was motivated by a theoretical issue—the interplay between transactions in the developmental ecology of adolescence and the larger stratification systems of American society—but was also purposely crafted, organized, and executed so as to connect this theoretical issue to extant policy aims and considerations.

Rather than studying learning or academic achievement (e.g., test performance, grades), I focused on course sequences—how adolescents move from one course to another over time. This focus provided one way to identify discrete stratifying events that schools can (and do) target in a systematic way (Crosnoe, 2009b).

Rather than concentrating on the kinds of emotional and psychological support that adolescents could derive from social relationships, I looked into how instrumental assistance—primarily in the form of concrete information and advice about how to navigate high school curricula to get to college—was traded through social ties. This approach was motivated by the perception that specific information deficits should be easier for in-school and out-of-school programs to address than differences in the more socioemotional aspects of relationships, such as closeness or emotional support (Crosnoe, 2009a).

Rather than studying friendships and cliques, which are difficult to manipulate through policy means, I examined peer influences among classmates and coursemates. These peer groupings, from which friendships and cliques often arise, are a function of school curricular organization, which has long been viewed as an appropriate venue of policy intervention (Crosnoe, Riegle-Crumb, Field, Frank, & Muller, 2008).

In taking these steps, I paid special attention to critical periods and groups of intervention, identifying points in the educational career and segments of the student population in which socioeconomic stratification was either particularly acute or particularly reactive to changes in social resources. For example, socioeconomic differences in the degree of slippage between middle school math status and high school math course enrollment, a root cause of socioeconomic disparities in end-of-school outcomes and college-going, were only found among low ability students (Crosnoe & Huston, 2007; Crosnoe & Schneider, 2010).

Finally, I employed a mixed methods strategy, integrating statistical analyses of national data sets that sketched out more causally robust population patterns with qualitative analyses of a single school to unpack the mechanisms at work. As described shortly, this approach allowed me to begin to address multiple demands of translational research (Crosnoe, 2011).

Overall, this body of research demonstrated not only that developmental and interpersonal considerations matter to educational inequality but also that these considerations have practical, not just theoretical, value. I followed a similar process in my other long-term projects, including investigations of the role of early childhood experiences in educational disparities related to Mexican immigration (Crosnoe, 2006) and of socioeconomic and gender differences in the impact of social marginalization in high school on college-going (Crosnoe, 2011). In both cases, I designed the study to focus on policy-relevant outcomes and predictors from the start, and, as a result, came up with answers that I thought could be important to major policy debates. I just had to get those answers out into the world beyond campus. My ongoing trial-and-error attempts to do so have given me several insights into how translational research works.

FOUR INSIGHTS ABOUT TRANSLATIONAL RESEARCH

Again, my qualification for writing about translational research is that I am a basic researcher slowly making my way toward translational research. I am not a fully formed translational researcher, at least not yet. Consequently, the insights that I share next are aimed at others like me, scholars (especially early career scholars) trained in traditional research-oriented programs who want to take what they are doing in a translational direction but face the daunting task of doing the hard work of this career change on their own. These insights are intended to help them avoid or deal with the early pitfalls in their endeavors that I myself faced.

Realistically Target a Level

Using research to inform policy is an awfully ambiguous (and ambitious) aim. After all, policy and related programmatic efforts play out on many different levels in both the public and private sectors. For many social and behavioral scientists outside of psychology, the policy domain is viewed in terms of the "big" policy debates surrounding federal and state legislation, such as welfare reform; the healthy marriage initiative; and, specifically, about education, No Child Left Behind and English-language learner support (Epstein, 2005; Furstenberg, 2007; Genesee, Lindholm-Leary, Saunders, & Christian, 2006; Sawhill, Weaver, Kane, & Haskins, 2002). Yet, given the scope of the policy activity involved and the stature of those involved in the debate, getting heard on these sweeping policy issues is quite difficult. One must have an "in," a platform—something few researchers, especially those early in their careers, have. Policy and related activities, however, also occur on a smaller scale, such as in local governments, nonprofit organizations, and extension services, and researchers may more easily forge partnerships with these smaller-scale efforts. Moreover, what they lack in profile, such activities make up for in immediate connections to peoples' lives.

When I began conducting my research on socioeconomic disparities in the path to college, I believed that I had something to add to national debates about educational policy, and although I was tapped into some professional networks that theoretically could have granted me access to the actors in those debates, I had no success in being heard. In some ways, however, I was lucky in that educational (and developmental) research has natural local units to which educational researchers interested in policy can connect—schools. I could change my policy orientation from the federal level to the local level, and I did so. The key is not to approach schools and school personnel with research findings tied to programmatic recommendations. Instead, as I explain in more detail below, it is to establish a relationship with schools through other means and let policy-oriented research emerge more organically from these relationships.

All of this is not to say that efforts to inform "big" policy are not worthwhile. They are, but they require a strategic plan and depend on social networks that need to be built and maintained. Researchers housed in policy programs within universities or in policy-oriented think tanks (e.g., the Brookings Institution) and those who have strong ties to either have an advantage in this regard over scholars housed in disciplinary departments at universities. For example, I have had more success getting my research on the education of immigrants to federal policymakers through my association with the Urban Institute, a Washington DC–based research institute, than through any ties I have had at my own university. In large part, this difference reflects the location of such institutes in federal and state capitals; the presence on staff of personnel with direct experience in government; the efficiency of contracted research that specifies efforts, products, and timetables; and the link between researchers and large support staffs (e.g., professional writers, publicists). Yet, the difference could also reflect that the researchers in these institutes have to be more agentic in their pursuit of converting basic research into translational research targeting the federal or state level, going beyond publishing articles in high-impact journals and then hoping that they reach a readership outside of academia.

Recognize the Power of "Voice"

In graduate school in a sociology department and in a postdoctoral fellowship at a population center, I was trained to view longitudinal statistical modeling of large representative data sets as a high standard of empirical evidence. Certainly, the rather traditional professional track I took in sociology and developmental psychology after securing my faculty position only reinforced this notion. The more sophisticated the methodology, the better the chances that an article would be published or a grant would be funded. Yet, when I began my attempts to use my research to inform policy, I was told repeatedly by established translational researchers and by those directly involved in policymaking that what mattered most was the bottom line conclusions; that sharing or delving into methodological detail and associated caveats, nuances, and contingencies would only be counterproductive; that people outside of academia had an inherent distrust of statistical modeling that undercut the message. "An anecdote from one kid will make more of a difference than a fancy quasi-experimental design any day," the dean of a school of education at a major state university (not my own) advised me. The implication is that solid empirical evidence requires a human voice to make an impact.

For me, one way around this disconnect between research training in universities and the reality of policy and intervention off campus is to use mixed method strategies, in which smaller scale and more personalized ethnographic and qualitative strategies are employed in a two-way exchange with larger-scale quantitative strategies (Duncan, Huston, & Weisner, 2007). This integrative approach provides the human voice in a rigorous, scientifically informed way and offers hard data in a form that diverse audiences want, not merely anecdotes.

For example, in my work on socioeconomic disparities in the path to college, I and my colleagues have applied a variety of statistical techniques to national-level longitudinal data to reveal causally robust patterns about how socioeconomically disadvantaged high school students get less—in the form of persistence in math or science coursework—from access to adult consultants (including parents) about their course enrollment decisions than their more advantaged peers. Our interpretation is that the explanation lies in socioeconomic differences in the quality of information about the steps to college being traded in social networks, not socioeconomic differences in values or social support (Crosnoe & Huston, 2007; Crosnoe & Schneider, 2010). In our view, these patterns and the conclusions to which they led spoke to some of the inadequacies of the family–school compact component of No Child Left Behind as well as in-school and out-of-school mentoring programs (Epstein, 2005; Spencer, 2006). In talking with school personnel about these findings, however, I was not able to gain any traction until I shared data from the linked school ethnography I had performed to identify the mechanisms underlying these statistical patterns. Consider the following comparison of two girls discussing their coursework decision-making process.

A low-socioecomic status (SES) girl opted to take a sign language class rather than advanced science because her mother, who desperately wanted her to go to college, figured that proving she was well-rounded would help her college-going chances and feared that a bad grade in a hard class might hurt her chances. "My mom is like, 'You just pick classes that . . . you might have a better chance of getting into college. So, I pick classes that college will look at . . . like clubs and language and art," she explained. Conversely, a high-SES girl opted to postpone taking sign language until the end of her senior year because her parents had advised her that she needed to fill her transcript with demanding courses to get into and not fail out of college. As she explained, "Taking core classes . . . that is what school is about. That's what you are there for. It would just kind of, I guess, defy the purpose of school [to do otherwise]." This comparison spoke to educators in a fundamental way. It provided voices that mattered to them.

Thus, by expanding my methodological toolkit, I was better able to unpack the quantitative results that seemed important to me and, as a side benefit, translate these results to diverse audiences. For both reasons, I now plan every major project as a quantitative–qualitative, national–local enterprise.

Utilize Both Sides of the Two-Way Relationship

From the perspective of a traditionally trained social and behavioral scientist, one of the hardest parts of translational research is understanding that the relationship between research and policy is not one way (researcher translating results to policymakers and practitioners) but instead two way (researcher translating results to policymakers and practitioners who are helping to guide the researcher's work, and so on). I think that my own personal experience—going into a policy setting with a research agenda and being less than open to suggestions and critiques from the audience—is likely indicative of a major obstacle to translational research. Our research is not the last word but instead a component of a much more complicated process (Cohen & Garet, 1975). Over time, I have become more open to the dialogue inherent to translational research.

On the one hand, engaging in an open dialogue with policymakers and practitioners helps researchers figure out what they need to study. More immersed in and in touch with the actual people subsumed within public health issues, social disparities, and so on, they have a better idea of important topics that are not well understood, and these ideas can be invigorating for researchers. For example, in working with local school district officials on a project about socioeconomic disparities in college-going, I was told about some of the pressing concerns of the district, including fades in achievement over time among low-income children who participated in the district's public pre-K program that may have been tied to differences in classroom quality across the transition from pre-K to kindergarten. Such conversations, which aligned well with the other work I was doing on early education and touched on ongoing debates in educational research (Brooks-Gunn, 2003), led me into a new mixed methods study on early classroom quality in at-risk populations that will mark a concerted partnership with the district on research.

On the other hand, an open dialogue also allows researchers to better convince nonresearch-oriented audiences about what their data say. After all, the same closeness to everyday process that enables practitioners to have a sense of pressing issues in need of study also might increase their reluctance to accept data-based conclusions that conflict with conventional wisdom or personal experience. In my own research, I found that school personnel, as well as parents, were often dismissive of the social concerns of adolescents until they saw data that demonstrated how the social ups and downs of high school life disrupted adolescents' trajectories into college and undermined major school reforms, such as mainstreaming and integration.

In short, translational relationships might be doomed to failure if researchers come in with the belief that they have scientific answers to enlighten practitioners and practitioners dismiss the input of researchers they see as divorced from "the real world" that they navigate every day. In any given relationship, the truth might lie in the middle or nearer to one side than the other. The challenge faced by translational researchers is to figure out, for any given partnership, where that balance is.

Understand the Culture

Often, researchers studying some policy-relevant educational or developmental issue are outsiders to the communities that are in the spotlight of their work. This is doubly so when they try to work with policymakers and practitioners in a research–policy partnership. This outsider status is a serious impediment to quality research and research-based practice for a variety of reasons, most of which center on cultural awareness or the lack thereof.

Without a good inside understanding of the focus of their research, social and behavioral scientists might lack key information needed to design the most effective studies, and they may misinterpret what they find, often in a deceptively negative light. At the same time, stakeholders might be suspicious (and dismissive) of scientists whom they view as too far removed from what they are studying. The burden is on researchers, therefore, to make good-faith efforts to familiarize themselves with the inner workings, and politics, of the programs, groups, organizations, and communities to which they hope to translate research.

The area in which I have most encountered these issues has been my research on the educational experiences of the children of Mexican immigrants (Crosnoe, 2006). This multiyear project, which drew primarily on quantitative data, was an example of basic research with an explicit agenda of informing policy, in this case early educational policy. Frequently, when meeting with both scholarly and public groups inside and outside university settings about this research, I was criticized, sometimes emotionally so, for reporting some findings (out of many) that appeared to cast Mexican immigrant families from a deficit perspective. This was clearly made more troubling by the fact that I was not of Mexican origins myself. How could I have any understanding of what Mexican immigrant families were like? Although the merits of this criticism can be (and were) respectfully argued, I realized quickly that the fact that these feelings were out there was a very real impediment to any goals I had about working with this community or the school serving this community to translate my research. Thus, I have reorganized the strategies I use to conduct this kind of research, incorporating Spanish-speaking, Mexican-origin students and colleagues into my projects, drawing on mixed methods strategies that require ample time "on the ground" with these communities, and starting with a dialogue in these communities about general research goals and working backward from there toward specific aims. Essentially, what I have done is anticipate the eventual challenges to translational research and, in the process, take steps to address them before they happen.

As further argument for the value of mixed methods approaches in translational research, they provide an effective way for researchers to teach themselves about the cultures of the groups they are studying or targeting and to self-correct as they face cultural barriers to effective translation. Having studied high schools for almost a decade with national-level secondary and primary data sources, not to mention having once been a high school student myself, I thought that I knew well how high schools and high school peer cultures worked. Yet, when I began the school ethnography component of my W. T. Grant and NICHD-funded projects on social relations in high schools, I was genuinely taken aback by how foreign everything seemed to me. The initial observations and interviews I conducted taught me, on the job, how to better conduct later observations and interviews, taught me the language I needed to use, the gatekeepers I needed to get on my side. Without this experience, the research on high schools that I was conducting, however sound it might have been, had a patina of inauthenticity that would not have made a difference in a journal publication but would have mattered a great deal in an applied setting.

One can believe that science should be free of the political struggles and cultural disconnects that cause strife in everyday life, but that belief does not preclude having to deal with such struggles and disconnects in conducting science. Indeed, they are basic facts of translational research, and the sooner that novice translational researchers learn this lesson the better.

CONCLUSION

Within the major disciplines of the social and behavioral sciences, debates often occur about the degree to which research in the discipline should play a role in public issues and, if so, what should that role be. When these debates occur, what is striking to me is not how much disagreement there is about these questions, nor the actual substance of the conversation. Instead, it is the fact there is any debate at all. Without much debate at all, large, vibrant disciplines should easily and supportively house scientists solely interested in basic research, those fully committed to applied or translational research, those wanting to go back and forth between the two models, and those wanting to be grounded in one but experiment with the other.

In truth, social and behavioral science disciplines do typically house all of this diversity, but they often do not equally or equitably support their diverse constituencies. Graduate students and young scholars who want to take a traditional basic research direction have many options. They can get training in what they want to do in any of the top programs, and their work will be appropriate for major journals and presses. The same is not true for graduate students and young scholars who want to go into a more public form of social and behavioral science, such as translational research. To get the training and support they need for this pursuit, they will have to be proactive, searching more widely and identifying specific programs and groups. Importantly, if basic research is the default setting for most prestigious departments in a discipline, any incoming student who does not yet know about translational research or is unsure about it will be unlikely to move in an applied direction. As a result, the discipline might lose potential translational researchers, thereby reinforcing the status quo. This phenomenon even plays out in disciplines that historically have had a highly public focus. Note, for example, the dialogues about the need for more scientific educational research surrounding the creation of the Institute of Education Sciences (Shavelson & Towne, 2006).

My own experience as a traditionally trained sociologist who is gradually moving toward a more public form of interdisciplinary science provides me a special perspective that is valuable in general discussions of translational research. I realize that these lessons are, for the most part, broad generalities. That is what happens with self-teaching. It is an idiosyncratic process that does not lend itself to universal yet specific advice. I also recognize that in discussing these lessons learned I run the risk of self-congratulation for very small steps when many of my colleagues across disciplines are doing so much more with their translational research. Yet, taking small steps is a natural function of the trial-and-error process that must occur when formal training is not easy to obtain; a product of the reality that a scientist grounded in a core social or behavioral science discipline often must balance translational pursuits with the other traditional activities demanded in those disciplines. In the end, however, I think that it is best to conceptualize such tensions as growing pains, a sign of slow but measurable change in a field of activity prone to inertia.

REFERENCES

Alexander, K. L., Entwisle, D., & Olson, L. S. (2007). Lasting consequences of the summer learning gap. *American Sociological Review, 72*, 167–180. doi:10.1177/000312240707200202

Arum, R. (2000). Schools and communities: Ecological and institutional dimensions. *Annual Review of Sociology, 26*, 395–418. doi:10.1146/annurev.soc.26.1.395

Attewell, P., & Domina, T. (2008). Raising the bar: Curricular intensity and academic performance. *Educational Evaluation and Policy Analysis, 30*, 51–71. doi:10.3102/0162373707313409

Barker, R., & Gump, P. V. (1964). *Big school, small school: High school size and student behavior*. Stanford, CA: Stanford University Press.

Bernhardt, A., Morris, M., Handcock, M. S., & Scott, M. A. (2001). *Divergent paths: Economic mobility in the new American labor market*. New York, NY: Russell Sage Foundation.

Bronfenbrenner, U., McClelland, P., Wethington, E., Moen, P., & Ceci, S. (1996). *The state of Americans: The disturbing facts and figures on changing values, crime, the economy, poverty, family, education, the aging population and what they mean for our future*. New York, NY: Free Press.

Brooks-Gunn, J. (2003). Do you believe in magic? What we can expect from early childhood intervention programs. *Society for Research in Child Development Social Policy Report, 17*(1), 3–14.

Cheadle, J. E. (2008). Educational investment, family context, and children's math and reading growth from kindergarten through third grade. *Sociology of Education, 81*, 1–31. doi:10.1177/003804070808100101

Chubb, J. E., & Moe, T. (1990). *Politics, markets, and American schools*. Washington, DC: Brookings Institution.

Clotfelter, C. T., Ladd, H. F., & Vigdor, J. (2007). Teacher credentials and student achievement: Longitudinal analysis with student fixed effects. *Economics of Education Review, 26*, 673–682. doi:10.1016/j.econedurev.2007.10.002

Cohen, D. K., & Garet, M. S. (1975). Reforming educational policy with applied research. *Harvard Educational Review, 45*(1), 17–43.

Crosnoe, R. (2001). Academic orientation and parental involvement in education during high school. *Sociology of Education, 74,* 210–230. doi:10.2307/2673275

Crosnoe, R. (2004). Social capital and the interplay of families and schools. *Journal of Marriage and Family, 66,* 267–280. doi:10.1111/j.1741-3737.2004.00019.x

Crosnoe, R. (2006). *Mexican roots, American schools: Helping Mexican immigrant children succeed.* Palo Alto, CA: Stanford University Press.

Crosnoe, R. (2009a). Family–school connections and the transitions of low-income youth and English language learners from middle school into high school. *Developmental Psychology, 45,* 1061–1076. doi:10.1037/a0016131

Crosnoe, R. (2009b). Low-income students and the socioeconomic composition of public high schools. *American Sociological Review, 74,* 709–730. doi:10.1177/000312240907400502

Crosnoe, R. (2011). *Fitting in, standing out, navigating the social challenges of high school to get an education.* New York, NY: Cambridge University Press.

Crosnoe, R., & Huston, A. C. (2007). Socioeconomic status, schooling, and the developmental trajectories of adolescents. *Developmental Psychology, 43,* 1097–1110. doi:10.1037/0012-1649.43.5.1097

Crosnoe, R., Riegle-Crumb, C., Field, S., Frank, K., & Muller, C. (2008). Peer contexts of girls' and boys' academic experiences. *Child Development, 79,* 139–155. doi:10.1111/j.1467-8624.2007.01116.x

Crosnoe, R., & Schneider, B. (2010). Social capital, information, and socioeconomic disparities in math coursework. *American Journal of Education, 117*(1), 79–107.

DiPrete, T. A., & Buchmann, C. (2006). Gender specific trends in the value of education and the emerging gender gap in college completion. *Demography, 43,* 1–24. doi:10.1353/dem.2006.0003

Domina, T. (2005). Leveling the home advantage: Assessing the effectiveness of parental involvement. *Sociology of Education, 78,* 233–249. doi:10.1177/003804070507800303

Dornbusch, S., Glasgow, K., & Lin, I. (1996). The social structure of schooling. *Annual Review of Psychology, 47,* 401–429. doi:10.1146/annurev.psych.47.1.401

Duncan, G. J., Huston, A. C., & Weisner, T. S. (2007). *Higher ground: New hope for the working poor and their children.* New York, NY: Russell Sage Foundation.

Epstein, J. L. (2005). Attainable goals? The spirit and letter of the No Child Left Behind Act on parental involvement. *Sociology of Education, 78,* 179–182. doi:10.1177/003804070507800207

Fischer, C. S., & Hout, M. (2006). *Century of difference: How America changed in the last one hundred years.* New York, NY: Russell Sage Foundation.

Fuller, B. (2007). *Standardized childhood: The political and cultural struggle over early education.* Palo Alto, CA: Stanford University Press.

Furstenberg, F. F. (2007). Should government promote marriage? *Journal of Policy Analysis and Management, 26,* 956–960. doi:10.1002/pam.20295

Gandara, P. (2002). A study of High School Puente: What we have learned about preparing Latino youth for postsecondary education. *Educational Policy, 16*, 474–495. doi:10.1177/0895904802164002

Genesee, F., Lindholm-Leary, K. J., Saunders, W., & Christian, D. (2006). *Educating English language learners.* New York, NY: Cambridge University Press. doi:10.1017/CBO9780511499913

Goldin, C., & Katz, L. F. (2008). *The race between technology and education.* Cambridge, MA: Harvard University Press.

Gormley, W. T., Gayer, T., Phillips, D., & Dawson, B. (2005). The effects of universal pre-k on cognitive development. *Developmental Psychology, 41*, 872–884. doi:10.1037/0012-1649.41.6.872

Heckman, J. J. (2006, June 30). Skill formation and the economics of investing in disadvantaged children. *Science, 312*, 1900–1902. doi:10.1126/science.1128898

Heckman, J. J., Lochner, L., & Todd, P. (2007). Earnings functions, rates of return and treatment effects: The Minder equation and beyond. In E. Hanushek & F. Welch (Eds.), *Handbook of the economics of education* (pp. 307–458). Amsterdam, The Netherlands: Elsevier.

Hill, N. E., & Tyson, D. (2009). Parental involvement in middle school: A meta-analytic assessment of the strategies that promote achievement. *Developmental Psychology, 45*, 740–763. doi:10.1037/a0015362

Hoxby, C. (2004). *College choices: The economics of where to go, when to go, and how to pay for it.* Chicago, IL: University of Chicago Press.

Huston, A. C. (2008). From research to policy and back. *Child Development, 79*, 1–12. doi:10.1111/j.1467-8624.2007.01107.x

Kane, T. (2007). Public intervention in postsecondary education. In E. Hanushek & F. Welch (Eds.), *Handbook of the economics of education* (pp. 1369–1402). Amsterdam, The Netherlands: Elsevier.

Karloy, L., Kilburn, M. R., & Cannon, J. S. (2006). *Early childhood interventions: Proven results, future promise.* Santa Monica, CA: Rand Corporation.

Knudsen, E. I., Heckman, J., Cameron, J., & Shonkoff, J. (2006). Economic, neurobiological, and behavioral perspectives on building America's future workforce. *Proceedings of the National Academy of Sciences of the United States of America, 103*, 10155–10162. doi:10.1073/pnas.0600888103

Lareau, A. (2004). *Unequal childhoods: Class, race, and family life.* Berkeley, CA: University of California Press.

Lee, V. E., & Ready, D. D. (2007). *Schools-within-schools: Possibilities and pitfalls of high school reform.* New York, NY: Teachers College Press.

Lemieux, T. (2006). Postsecondary education and increased wage inequality. *The American Economic Review, 96*, 195–199. doi:10.1257/000282806777211667

Love, J. M., Kisker, E., Ross, C., Raikes, H., Constantine, J., Boller, K., . . . Vogel, C. (2005). The effectiveness of Early Head Start for 3-year-old children and their parents: Lesson for policy and programs. *Developmental Psychology, 41*, 885–901. doi:10.1037/0012-1649.41.6.885

Ludwig, J., & Sawhill, I. (2007). *Success by ten: Intervention early, often, and effectively in the education of young children*. Washington, DC: Brookings Institution Press.

Massey, D. S. (1996). The age of extremes: Concentrated affluence and poverty in the Twenty First Century. *Demography, 33*, 395–412. doi:10.2307/2061773

Morgan, S. L. (2005). *On the edge of commitment: Educational attainment and race in the United States*. Stanford, CA: Stanford University Press.

National Commission on Excellence in Education. (1983). *A nation at risk: The imperative for educational reform*. Washington, DC: U.S. Department of Education.

Pianta, R. C., Cox, M. J., & Snow, K. L. (2007). *School readiness and the transition to kindergarten in the era of accountability*. Baltimore, MD: Brookes.

Raver, C. C., Jones, S. M., Li-Grining, C., Metzger, M., Smallwood, K., & Sardin, L. (2008). Improving preschool classroom processes: Preliminary findings from a randomized trial implemented in Head Start settings. *Early Childhood Research Quarterly, 63*, 10–26. doi:10.1016/j.ecresq.2007.09.001

Sabir, M., Breckman, R., Meador, R., Wethington, E., Reid, M. C., & Pillemer, K. (2006). The CITRA research-practice consensus-workshop model: Exploring a new method of research translation in aging. *The Gerontologist, 46*, 833–839. doi:10.1093/geront/46.6.833

Sadler, P. M., & Tai, R. H. (2007, July 27). The two high school pillars supporting college sciences. *Science, 317*, 457–458. doi:10.1126/science.1144214

Sawhill, I., Weaver, K., Kane, A., & Haskins, R. (Eds.). (2002). *Welfare reform and beyond*. Washington, DC: Bookings Institution Press.

Schneider, B. S. (2007). *Forming a college-going community in U.S. schools*. Seattle, WA: Bill and Melinda Gates Foundation.

Shavelson, R., & Towne, L. (2002). *Scientific research in education*. Washington, DC: National Academy Press.

Spencer, R. (2006). Understanding the mentoring process between adolescents and adults. *Youth & Society, 37*, 287–315. doi:10.1177/0743558405278263

Swail, W. S., & Perna, L. W. (2002). Pre-college outreach programs: A national perspective. In W. G. Tierney & L. S. Hagedorn (Eds.), *Increasing access to college: Extending possibilities for all students* (pp. 15–34). Albany, NY: SUNY Press.

Tierney, W. G., Bailey, T., Constantine, J., Finkelstein, N., Hurd, N. F., Max, J., & Tuttle, C. C. (2009). *Helping students navigate the path to college: What high schools can do* (NCEE Report No. 2009-4066). Washington, DC: U. S. Department of Education, National Center for Educational Evaluation.

Turner, S., & Bound, J. (2006). *Cohort crowding: How resources affect collegiate attainment*. National Bureau of Economic Research Working Paper Series 12424.

Woolf, S. (2008). The meaning of translational research and why it matters. *JAMA, 299*, 211–213. doi:10.1001/jama.2007.26

4

A SYSTEMATIC REVIEW OF HEALTH PROMOTION AND DISEASE PREVENTION PROGRAM ADAPTATIONS: HOW ARE PROGRAMS ADAPTED?

LUDMILA N. KRIVITSKY, SAMANTHA J. PARKER, ANUSMIRITI PAL, LEIGH MECKLER, ROUZI SHENGELIA, AND M. CARRINGTON REID

Improvements in access to and implementation of evidence-based treatments are a principal goal of translational research, particularly in the health service and public health fields (Woolf, 2008). Just as there has been a push, notably from the National Institutes of Health, to improve translational research in biomedical and human service fields, the evidence-based practice movement has grown steadily over the past 2 decades. Numerous efforts and initiatives have been undertaken to promote the diffusion of evidence-based programs (EBPs) into diverse practice settings. The Social Work Policy Institute (2010) provides a comprehensive listing of registries and databases of evidence-based research, with a focus on social justice, child welfare, mental health, and substance abuse treatment and prevention. The Administration on Aging's (2010) Evidence-Based Disease and Disability Prevention Program seeks to increase older adults' access to EBPs with the goal of reducing their risk of injury, disability, or disease. In addition, the Substance Abuse and Mental

This research project was supported by a grant from the National Institute of Nursing Research (R21 NR010200-03). Additional support was provided by the National Institute on Aging: An Edward R. Roybal Center Grant (P30 AG022845-07) and the John A. Hartford Foundation.

Health Services Administration has developed and maintains the National Registry of Evidence-Based Programs and Practices. This searchable online registry contains information on more than 160 evidence-based substance abuse and mental health programs (U.S. Department of Health and Human Services, 2010). Finally, the Centers for Disease Control and Prevention (CDC) funded the Diffusion of Effective Behavioral Interventions project in 1999 to promote the diffusion of evidence-based HIV prevention programs via community-based organizations, as well as state and local health departments (Diffusion of Effective Behavioral Interventions, 2010).

The goal of T3 translational research is to overcome barriers that prevent broad dissemination of best practices from research institutions to community practice (Westfall, Mold, & Fagnan, 2007). There are many such barriers, not the least of which is an insufficiency of resources to implement complex interventions at the agency level. In addition, organizations may seek to implement an EBP in a population that differs culturally, geographically, or with respect to risk behaviors or age composition from the population that was employed to establish the program's effectiveness. Finally, stakeholders in the new setting in which the EBP will be implemented may demand program changes to achieve buy-in prior to implementation. To reduce the cost or accommodate differences between the populations employed to develop and test the original intervention versus new target populations, EBPs frequently require adaptation. Indeed, research that has examined the diffusion of EBPs in practice has documented that program adaptation is typically the rule rather than the exception (Galbraith, 2004). In a review of 34 agencies that implemented Focus on Kids, an evidence-based HIV prevention program (Galbraith et al., 1996), Galbraith (2004) demonstrated that all but one of the agencies made changes to the curriculum, including program deletions and additions.

Making changes to improve a program's "fit" in a given community raises several important questions. What types of information should be gathered to determine the types of changes needed for implementation? Once this information is collected, how will the information be translated into actual program modifications? Who will be responsible for making the changes? What types of changes are acceptable? While certain adaptations may enhance a program's fit, how frequently do changes lead to a decrease in program effectiveness because an essential component has been changed? Should the adapted program be compared with the original program in the new target population to establish equivalence in terms of outcomes?

At least six published guidelines provide specific recommendations regarding the steps that should be taken to adapt EBPs and may help to address some of the above questions (Backer, 2002; Kumpfer, Pinyuchon, Texieria de Melo, & Whiteside, 2008; Lee, Altschul, & Mowbray, 2008; McKleroy et al., 2006; Smith & Caldwell, 2007; Wingood & DiClemente, 2008). Table 4.1

TABLE 4.1

Program Adaptation Guideline Summaries[a]

Backer (2002)	Kumpfer et al. (2008)	Lee et al. (2008)	McKleroy et al. (2006)	Smith and Caldwell (2007)	Wingood and DiClemente (2008)
1. Understand theory behind program[b]	1. Generate needs assessment data on etiological precursors of target condition	1. Determine whether EBP has discernible theory of change; core components responsible for change should not be modified[b]	1. Assess: Ascertain behavioral determinants and risk behaviors of new target population; identify one or more relevant EBPs; identify core program elements; identify core program elements; identify areas where EBP needs to be adapted[b]; seek input from advisory boards and community planning groups; assess organizational capacity to implement program	1. Determine potential differences in new target setting versus setting in which program was originally developed	1. Assessment: Conduct focus groups, interviews, needs assessments with new target population; assess agency capacity
2. Locate or conduct core component analysis of program	2. Select EBP deemed most appropriate for new target population[b]	2. Determine how original and new target population differ	2. Select: Pick EBP and decide whether to adapt or implement original program; determine which changes are needed and make them; consult content experts as needed	2. Determine whether developmental processes in original and new target populations differ	2. Decision: Review relevant EBPs; decide on most appropriate program for new setting and determine whether program requires adaptation[b]

(continues)

TABLE 4.1
Program Adaptation Guideline Summaries[a]   *(Continued)*

Backer (2002)	Kumpfer et al. (2008)	Lee et al. (2008)	McKleroy et al. (2006)	Smith and Caldwell (2007)	Wingood and DiClemente (2008)
3. Assess fidelity and adaptation concerns for target site; determine what adaptations may be necessary	3. Pilot test EBP in new target population	3. Adapt program contents through collaborative efforts	3. Prepare: Train staff, pretest adapted materials with stakeholder groups	3. Determine whether differences exist in risk and protective factors between new and original target populations	3. Administration: Theater test selected EBP using new target population and other stakeholders to generate adaptations
4. Consult original program developers as needed	4. Select and train staff to ensure quality implementation	4. Evaluate adapted program and include instruments to assess effects of the new program components	4. Pilot: Develop implementation plan and conduct pilot test of adapted EBP; modify EBP further if necessary	4. Determine level of program adaptation needed to include possible changes in program structure, content, provider or delivery methods	4. Production: Adapt EBP maintaining fidelity to core elements; develop adaptation plan
5. Consult with stakeholders where program implementation will take place	5. Implement program		5. Implement: Execute adapted EBP	5. Consider phased process of program dissemination (allowing for pilot testing); attend to issues of program sustainability	5. Topical experts: Obtain input from experts in field

6. Develop implementation plan based on results generated in above steps	6. Make cultural adaptations continuously through pilot testing 7. Revise program based on results generated in step 6 8. Employ participatory research and empowerment evaluation approach framework to improve program implementation 9. Disseminate results	6. Identify stakeholder partners who can champion program adoption in new setting and ensure program fidelity	6. Integration: Incorporate expert advice into program; conduct readability tests 7. Training: Train staff 8. Testing: Pilot test adapted program

Note. EBP = evidence-based program.
[a]Guidelines focused on adapting HIV/sexually transmitted disease prevention programs (McKleroy et al., 2006; Wingood & DiClemente, 2008), substance abuse programs (Backer, 2002), the Strengthening Families Program (Kumpfer et al., 2008), or on adapting general health promotion–disease prevention programs (Lee et al., 2008; Smith & Caldwell, 2007).
[b]Literature review was part of adaptation step.

summarizes the adaptation steps present in the six guidelines. A review of the recommendations reveals substantial interguideline differences. For example, with respect to the types of information that should be obtained in preparation for program adaptation, four of the six include a needs assessment step as a means of generating information to inform the adaptation process, whereas three recommend that content experts be consulted. Only two of the guidelines (Kumpfer et al., 2008; Wingood & DiClemente, 2008) provide detailed recommendations regarding strategies for generating suggested program adaptations. For example, Wingood and DiClemente (2008) recommended pretesting specific modules of the EBP (but not the entire program) with small groups composed of the new target population. The evaluation is followed by a survey and a group discussion with participants, as well as other stakeholders, including agency staff. Both sets of data are then used to inform the adaptation process.

With respect to the types of programmatic changes that are permissible, all six guidelines uniformly recommend that no changes be made to core programmatic elements. These core elements are defined by CDC as "components that are critical features of an intervention intent and design and are thought to be responsible for its effectiveness" (Wingood & DiClemente, 2008, p. S43). These components can be identified through scientific component analysis conducted by the program developer or the program implementer (Backer, 2002), or by closely examining the theoretical basis of the intervention, as suggested by Wingood and DiClemente (2008) and by Lee et al. (2008).

Indeed, Wingood and DiClemente (2008) defined adaptation not just as any change or modification to the original program but as a "process of modifying an evidence-based program without competing or contradicting its core elements or internal logic" (p. S40). Similarly, McKleroy et al. (2006) referred to adaptation as "the process of modifying key characteristics of an intervention, recommended activities and delivery methods, without competing with or contradicting the core elements, theory, and internal logic of the intervention" (p. 62). These definitions highlight an essential tension that often exists during the adaptation process, that is, the need to maintain fidelity to core elements while simultaneously recognizing the need to modify program components to maximize program fit for a new target population (Castro, Barrera, & Martinez, 2004).

At present, limited information exists regarding T3 translational research methodologies employed to modify EBPs so that they are more appropriate for dissemination among diverse populations and settings. Filling this knowledge gap would allow potential program adapters to learn about methodologies used by groups in other communities and could pave the way for identifying optimal adaptation methodologies. We therefore conducted a systematic review of English-language articles to determine the types of adaptation approaches used (and corresponding types of adaptations made) in studies that reported data on these outcomes. An additional objective was to determine whether studies employed any of the six guidelines listed in Table 4.1 during the adaptation process. Finally, given uniform agreement with regard to the recommendation to avoid changes to core programmatic components (see the guideline summaries in Table 4.1), we determined the frequency with which articles adhered to this recommendation.

METHOD

Data Sources and Searches

We searched the PubMed/Medline, Embase, PsycINFO, and Web of Science databases from January 1999 through March 2010. Specific Medical Subject Headings (MeSH) terms included *health promotion, community health planning,* and *delivery of healthcare.* Other search terms included *program development, health program, community program, voluntary program, community health,* and *public health.* These terms and the PubMed MeSH terms were then combined with the following search words: *adapt, modify, tailor,* and *translate.*

Study Selection

Abstracts identified in the searches were reviewed in detail by at least two authors. Abstracts suggesting that program adaptation was the goal of the study were retained, and the full text of each article was reviewed by two authors. To be eligible for inclusion in the review, studies had to be published in English and state that a goal of the investigation was either to (a) adapt an evidence-based health promotion or disease prevention program or to (b) evaluate an adapted program *and* provide information regarding the approach used for program adaptation. The reference lists of all retained articles were reviewed to identify other potentially suitable studies. The search strategy generated 15,656 abstracts, which were reviewed by two investigators (AP, SJP). The most common reasons for excluding abstracts were the following: (a) did not report on the adaptation of a health promotion or disease prevention program ($n = 9,432$), (b) were duplicate studies ($n = 5,203$), (c) were review articles ($n = 679$), or (d) were published in a language other than English ($n = 180$). A total of 162 full-text articles were reviewed in detail; 125 were excluded. Common exclusions included articles that were methodological and did not present primary data ($n = 25$), described the evaluation of the adapted program only ($n = 22$), characterized the adaptation of a program that was not focused on health promotion ($n = 19$), described the creation of a completely new program ($n = 18$), or presented results from an effectiveness study ($n = 18$). Twenty-three articles were excluded for other reasons. This resulted in a final sample of 37 articles.

Study Outcomes

Two authors (LK, SJP) abstracted the following information from each retained article: (a) type of program adapted, (b) target population for the adapted program, (c) methods used to adapt the program, (d) adaptations made to the original program, and (e) whether studies employed one of the published guidelines listed in Table 4.1 during the adaptation process. Finally, we determined the frequency with which articles adhered to the key recommendation present in all six guidelines, that is, to avoid making changes to core programmatic components.

Additional outcomes of interest included the time required to complete the adaptation process and whether investigators employed community-based participatory research (CBPR) methods. We collected information on use of CBPR methods because several adaptation guidelines (Kumpfer et al., 2008; Wingood & DiClemente, 2008) recommend using this approach throughout the research process.

Because a primary goal of the current study was to catalogue the types of adaptation approaches employed, we critically reviewed each article and recorded all of the steps used in the process. Two investigators (LK, SJP) independently reviewed each article to identify the processes used and then met to review their results. Disagreements generally arose when there was insufficient information present in the article. The investigators resolved all coding differences through discussion.

A key additional goal was to identify the specific types of adaptations reported. Three papers (Backer, 2002; Castro et al., 2004; Smith & Caldwell, 2007) provided guidance for the classification system used in this study. Categories presented in these three papers include program structure, content, and provider (program administrator) or delivery (Smith & Caldwell, 2007) methods; modifications to program content or delivery style (Backer, 2002; Castro et al., 2004); changes to the core program components, cultural changes, and changes to the intensity of program administration (Backer, 2002). Two investigators (LK, SJP) independently abstracted details regarding the types of adaptations present in each article. All of the investigators (LK, SJP, AP, LM, RS, MCR) reviewed these results and determined that the reported adaptations could be organized into one of four distinct categories: (a) content additions, (b) changes in delivery, (c) cosmetic changes, or (d) content deletions. We also attempted to categorize the first three types of adaptations (content additions, delivery changes, and content deletions) as either cultural or noncultural. However, in many cases it was not possible to determine whether a given adaptation was motivated by cultural differences in the target population relative to the population tested in the development of the original program. After finalizing the classification system, two primary abstractors (LK, SJP) placed each article's abstracted adaptations into one of the four mutually exclusive categories, met to compare their results, and resolved all differences in coding through discussion.

RESULTS

Target Populations and Conditions

Most articles in the study (95%) reported making adaptations to EBPs for new target populations, such as a program originally developed for use by older adults in the United States that was subsequently adapted for older adults in the Netherlands (Zijlstra, Tennstedt, van Haastregt, Kempen, & van Eijk, 2006). The remaining two articles did not specify a change in target population but instead adapted the programs' method of delivery (e.g., adapted a community-based program for use as an online program).

Table 4.2 shows the types of programs adapted by disease category. The most prevalent studies identified were those adapting programs designed to reduce the spread of HIV or improve treatment adherence for HIV and other STDs. Other program types included substance abuse and misuse, chronic disease management, and mental health.

Types of EBP Adaptations

Program adaptations were grouped into one of the following four categories: (a) *content additions*, defined as an addition to the program (e.g., adding exercise to a program that did not have an exercise component) or enhancement of an existing program (e.g., increasing the amount of exercise in a program that already had an exercise component); (b) *changes in delivery*, defined as a change in an aspect of how, where, or by whom the program was actually delivered; (c) *cosmetic changes*, defined as a superficial program change, such as renaming the program; and (d) *content deletions*, defined as removal of a program component or abridgment of existing materials.

Content additions to include content enhancements were described in 31 articles (84%). For example, Quinn et al. (2006) added two booklets to the curriculum in a booklet-based smoking relapse prevention program adapted for pregnant and postpartum women: one targeting the woman's partner and one strategically timed for the baby's arrival. Tsarouk, Thompson, Herting, Walsh, and Randell (2007) provided an example of a content

TABLE 4.2

Characteristics of Study Sample

First author (Date)	Original program	Target population for adapted program[a]	Adaptation processes	Types of adaptations
		HIV/STD programs		
Copenhaver (2009)	Holistic Health Recovery Program	HIV-infected prisoners transitioning from prison to community	Conducted literature review, conducted needs assessment	Delivery Cosmetic Content deletions
Cornelius (2008)	Sisters Informing Sisters on Topics About AIDS	Older (50+ years old) African American women	Obtained direct feedback regarding original program from stakeholder group(s)	Content additions Delivery Cosmetic
Wainberg (2007)	Combined components from 6 evidence-based HIV prevention programs[b]	Psychiatric patients in Brazil	Conducted literature review, conducted needs assessment, described method used to translate suggested program modifications into actual adaptations, evaluated adapted program	Content additions Delivery Cosmetic
Devieux (2004)	Cognitive–Behavioral Stress Management Program	HIV-infected individuals in Haiti	Evaluated adapted program	Content additions Cosmetic
Lerdboon (2008)	Vietnamese Focus on Kids	Young males and females (15–21 years old) in Vietnam	Conducted needs assessment, evaluated adapted program	Content additions Delivery Cosmetic
Somerville (2006)	Popular Opinion Leader Program and components from 4 other evidence-based programs[b]	Young Latino migrant males	Conducted needs assessment, evaluated adapted program	Content additions Delivery Cosmetic
Fiscian (2009)	Making Proud Choices	Adolescent (10–17 years old) girls in Ghana	Conducted needs assessment, evaluated adapted program	Content additions Delivery Cosmetic Content deletions

Hitt (2006)	Project RESPECT-2	Persons receiving HIV counseling, testing, and referral services	Obtained direct feedback regarding original program from stakeholder group(s)	Content additions Delivery
Li (2006)	Voluntary Counseling & Testing Program	Female sex workers in China	Not described	Content additions Delivery
Mueller (2009)	¡Cuidate!	Latino urban high school students	Obtained input from content expert(s), evaluated adapted program	Content additions Delivery Content deletion
Wegner (2008)	(a) Life Skills Training (b) Time Wise: Taking Charge of Leisure Time (c) Sexuality curricula employed but not named	Adolescent and high school students in South Africa	Conducted literature review, evaluated adapted program	Content additions Delivery Cosmetic Content deletions
NIMH (2007)[c]	Community Popular Opinion Leader	Communities in China, India, Peru, Russia, and Zimbabwe	Conducted needs assessment, obtained direct feedback regarding original program from stakeholder group(s), evaluated adapted program	Content additions
Bhana (2004)	Collaborative HIV/AIDS & Adolescent Mental Health Programme	Families in South Africa	Conducted needs assessment, evaluated adapted program	Content additions Delivery Cosmetic
Villarruel (2005)	Be Proud! Be Responsible!	Latino adolescents	Conducted literature review, conducted needs assessment, obtained direct feedback regarding original program from stakeholder group(s), evaluated adapted program	Content additions Cosmetic

(continues)

TABLE 4.2
Characteristics of Study Sample   *(Continued)*

First author (Date)	Original program	Target population for adapted program[a]	Adaptation processes	Types of adaptations
			Substance abuse	
Steiker (2008)	Keepin' It Real	High-risk adolescents (14–19 years old) in community settings	Obtained direct feedback regarding original program from stakeholder group(s)	Content additions Cosmetic Content deletions
Tsarouk (2007)	Reconnecting Youth Drug Prevention Program	Adolescents (14–20 years old) in Russia with poor school performance	Obtained direct feedback regarding original program from stakeholder group(s), evaluated adapted program	Content additions Cosmetic Content deletions
Rey (2007)	Family Alcohol Intervention Program	Indigenous families in central Mexico	Conducted needs assessment, obtained direct feedback regarding original program from stakeholder group(s)	Cosmetic
Komro (2004)	Project Northland	Ethnically and racially diverse populations of urban youth	Conducted literature review, conducted needs assessment, obtained direct feedback regarding original program from stakeholder group(s), described method used to translate suggested program modifications into actual adaptations, evaluated adapted program	Content additions Delivery Cosmetic
Quinn (2006)	Forever Free Relapse Prevention Program	Pregnant and post-partum women	Conducted literature review, conducted needs assessment, obtained direct feedback regarding original program from stakeholder group(s), evaluated adapted program	Content additions

Sarkisian (2005)	Self-Care Empowerment Curriculum	Older African Americans and Latinos with diabetes	Conducted needs assessment, obtained direct feedback regarding original program from stakeholder group(s)	Content additions Delivery
Walker (2005)	Chronic Disease Self-Management Program	Minority communities (Vietnamese, Greek, Chinese, Italian) living in Australia	Conducted needs assessment, obtained direct feedback regarding original program from stakeholder group(s)	Cosmetic
Gitlin (2008)	Chronic Disease Self-Management Program	Older African Americans attending senior centers	Conducted needs assessment, obtained direct feedback regarding original program from stakeholder group(s), evaluated adapted program	Content additions Delivery Cosmetic
Punzalan (2006)	Diabetes Prevention Program	Low-income African American and Latino communities	Conducted needs assessment, evaluated adapted program	Content additions Delivery
McTigue (2009)	Diabetes Prevention Program	Individuals with elevated ($\geq$ 25) body mass index and cardiovascular risk factors	Obtained input from content expert(s), evaluated adapted program	Delivery
Ackermann (2007)	Diabetes Prevention Program	Individuals attending YMCAs	Not described	Content additions Delivery Cosmetic Content deletions
Belansky (2006)	Integrated Nutrition Education Program	Elementary school students in rural community	Obtained direct feedback regarding original program from stakeholder group(s), evaluated adapted program	Content additions Delivery
Reijneveld (2003)	Healthy & Vital	Older Turkish adults residing in the Netherlands	Conducted literature review, conducted needs assessment, obtained input from content expert(s), obtained direct feedback regarding original program from stakeholder group(s), evaluated adapted program	Content additions Delivery Cosmetic Content deletions

(continues)

TABLE 4.2

Characteristics of Study Sample *(Continued)*

First author (Date)	Original program	Target population for adapted program[a]	Adaptation processes	Types of adaptations
Karanja (2002)	Freedom from Fat[d]	African American women	Conducted literature review, conducted needs assessment, evaluated adapted program	Delivery Cosmetic
Pekmezi (2009)	Jump Start to Health	Overweight/ obese Latina/ Hispanic women with low income and acculturation	Conducted needs assessment, evaluated adapted program	Content additions Cosmetic
Zijlstra (2006)	A Matter of Balance	Community-dwelling older adults residing in the Netherlands	Obtained input from content expert(s), described method used to translate suggested program modifications into actual adaptations, evaluated adapted program	Content additions Delivery Cosmetic Content deletions
Mental health				
Kataoka (2006)	Cognitive–Behavioral Intervention for Trauma in Schools	Latino students attending parochial school	Conducted needs assessment, obtained direct feedback regarding original program from stakeholder group(s)	Content additions Delivery
Kanowski (2009)	Mental Health First Aid	Aboriginal peoples in Australia	Obtained direct feedback regarding original program from stakeholder group(s), obtained input from content expert(s), evaluated adapted program	Content additions Delivery Cosmetic
D'Angelo (2009)	Beardslee Preventive Intervention Program for Depression	Low-income Latino families	Conducted literature review, conducted needs assessment, obtained direct feedback regarding original program from stakeholder group(s), evaluated adapted program	Content additions Delivery

Study	Program	Target population	Other	Modifications
McIntyre (2008)	Incredible Years Parent Training	Parents of small children (2–5 years old) with developmental delay	Obtained direct feedback regarding original program from stakeholder group(s), evaluated adapted program	Content additions Cosmetic Content deletions
Marek (2006)	Strengthening Families Program	Families with young children (6–10 years old)	Conducted literature review, obtained direct feedback regarding original program from stakeholder group(s), evaluated adapted program	Content additions Delivery Cosmetic Content deletions
Tsey (2005)	Family Wellbeing Empowerment	Students (9–12 years old) from indigenous Australian communities	Evaluated adapted program	Content additions Delivery
Burgio (2009)	Resources for Enhancing Alzheimer's Caregiver Health II Program	Dementia caregivers	Obtained direct feedback regarding original program from stakeholder group(s), evaluated adapted program	Content deletions Delivery

aUnless specified, study was conducted in the United States. bThe authors reported adapting elements from evidence-based HIV prevention programs; however, the programs were not reported. cThree National Institute of Mental Health papers published sequentially to describe the adaptation project (National Institute of Mental Health Collaborative HIV/STD Prevention Trial Group (2007a, 2007b, 2007c). dGroup utilized the Freedom from Fat program's nutrition component only.

enhancement in their adaptation of a drug use prevention program for use by at-risk teenagers in Russia. During the adaptation process, a component of the original program in which teenagers were asked to share personal experiences or impressions was changed to a less personal, more abstract discussion. This change was made because Russian youth were perceived to be less accustomed to divulging personal feelings in a group setting than American teenagers.

Twenty-seven articles (73%) described making program delivery changes, which consisted of changes in the way intervention content was conveyed, without making changes to the program's content. Specific examples included converting a one-on-one intervention format to a group-based format, changing the qualifications required of the person(s) implementing the program, expanding or condensing the duration of the intervention without adding or removing content, changing the type of facility in which the intervention was held, and changing the mode of presentation.

Cosmetic changes were described in 24 articles (65%) and involved changes in either language or the use of cultural references. Most cosmetic changes involved changing the name of the program. For example, Cornelius, Moneyham, and LeGrand (2008) changed the name of an HIV prevention program targeting young women, "Sisters Informing Sisters on Topics About AIDS," to "Women Informing Women on Topics About AIDS" to make it more appropriate for use by older African American women (the new target population). In another cosmetic change in the same study, the term *boyfriend* was replaced by *partner, significant other*, or *friend*.

Finally, 12 articles (32%) reported making content deletions. Reijneveld, Westhoff, and Hopman-Rock (2003) adapted a health education and physical activity promotion program for use by older Turkish immigrants in the Netherlands. Focus group participants suggested that bicycling not be included as an example of physical exercise (a recommendation that was present in the original program) because bicycling was an uncommon means of exercising in the target population.

Processes and Time Frames for Adapting EBPs

Eleven studies (30%) employed CBPR methods. For example, six studies (16%) assembled a community advisory committee to oversee all aspects of the adaptation process. Seventeen studies (43%) reported time frames for completing their adaptations. The average time required to adapt an EBP was 2.5 years (range = 1–5 years). In most cases, this interval included conducting an evaluation of the adapted program.

We identified six distinct methods that investigators used to adapt EBPs (Figure 4.1), including performing literature reviews, consulting content

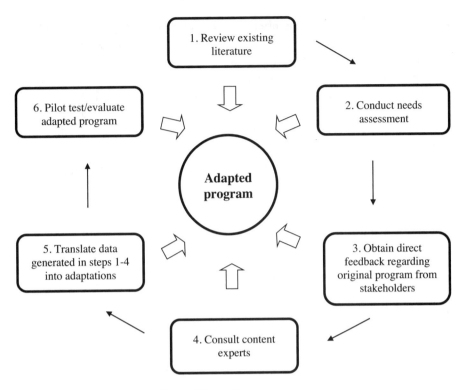

Figure 4.1. Steps used to adapt evidence-based programs.

experts, and evaluating the adapted program to generate additional program changes. No study reported using all six adaptation steps, and most (65%) used two or fewer steps; eight studies did not report using any steps. The mean number of steps employed was 2.3 (*Mdn* = 2; range = 0–4 steps). The following paragraphs describe the adaptation steps used and an example of each.

Ten studies (27%) performed literature reviews to help select EBPs or to review the content of selected EBPs or target population characteristics. In most cases, the literature review was the first step in the adaptation process. For example, to adapt an HIV risk-reduction intervention for use by HIV-infected prisoners about to transition to the community, Copenhaver, Chowdhury, and Altice (2009) reviewed existing EBPs to select the most appropriate intervention for their target population.

Twenty studies (54%) conducted a needs assessment as part of the adaptation process by collecting primary data from the target population or other stakeholders, such as community leaders. Primary data collection tools in these assessments included focus groups (80%) and survey methods, such as in-person interviews and questionnaires (73%). For example, D'Angelo et al. (2009) interviewed members of the target population regarding their beliefs about depression and resilience to adapt the Preventive Intervention Program for Depression program for use by low-income Latino families.

Nineteen studies (51%) obtained direct feedback about the original program from various stakeholder groups. Focus group methods were used by most studies (76%) to obtain feedback. The original program was described, and focus group participants were asked to provide suggestions regarding how best to adapt the program for optimal use by the target population. For example, Sarkisian et al. (2005) adapted a diabetes management intervention for use by older African Americans and Latinos by convening focus groups with members of the target population, describing the original program to participants, and asking them to suggest modifications. In the five remaining studies that employed this method, participants took part in the complete (unadapted) program and offered feedback regarding ways to improve the program for use by the new target population.

A few studies (14%) used content experts that included specialists or authorities with knowledge about the target condition, the target population, or the intervention itself. For example, in a study to adapt an American program to reduce the fear of falling among older adults living in the Netherlands, Dutch experts in geriatrics and gerontology were asked to review a translated version of the program and consulted the program administrators about implementation factors such as eligibility criteria for participation, facilitator qualifications, and appropriateness of the content for the new target population (Zijlstra et al., 2006).

While all of the studies used various methods to generate possible program changes and then incorporated some of the suggested recommendations into actual adaptations, only three (8%) reported an explicit method, that is, a "translation" step that was used to adjudicate suggested recommendations and incorporate them into the program. For example, to translate ethnographic data and prevention priorities into changes to an HIV prevention program, Wainberg et al. (2007) created an intervention adaptation work group comprising stakeholders and content experts. The work group and research team met three times to discuss adapting program content. At the meetings, the group determined the relevance, cultural appropriateness, and feasibility of implementing each recommendation; decided which content areas would be retained, modified, removed, or replaced; determined the order and location of program changes; and practiced and refined program exercises and the program.

Twenty-seven articles (73%) reported an evaluation of the adapted program. In most cases, evaluations consisted of piloting the adapted intervention with the target population and obtaining feedback. For example, an evidence-based parenting skills program for parents of children without developmental delays was adapted for use by parents of developmentally delayed children. The adapted program was piloted, feedback was solicited from participants, and the program was revised using these data (McIntyre, 2008). Ten articles (36%) examined the potential benefit of the adapted program in relation to a comparison group, which included participants who experienced the original health program, a similar health program, or usual care. For example, Reijneveld et al. (2003) tested an adapted chronic disease management intervention against a control health program, whereas Li et al. (2006) tested an adapted STD/HIV counseling and testing program in relation to usual care for STD testing and treatment.

Use of and Adherence to Published Guideline Recommendations

Only one study cited use of a published adaptation guideline. Copenhaver et al. (2009) employed Wingood and DiClemente's ADAPT-ITT model (see Table 4.1 for details) as a guide during the adaptation of an intervention targeting HIV-infected prisoners about to transition to the community. Finally, 14 studies (38%) adhered to the key recommendation that core elements of the original program be maintained, with the authors explicitly stating that core program components were not modified during the adaptation process.

DISCUSSION

This study adds to the nascent literature on program adaptation by demonstrating that diverse approaches have been employed to adapt EBPs over the past decade to include performing literature reviews, conducting needs assessments, and undertaking evaluations of the adapted programs as a means of generating additional program revisions. Studies reported using an average of 2.3 discrete adaptation steps out of the six possible. An analysis of the various approaches taken by the 37 studies revealed no predominant pattern. The adaptation initiatives took, on average, 2.5 years to complete, while one took 5 years. These numbers demonstrate that program adaptation is a time- and labor-intensive process, and raise significant questions about the feasibility of conducting this type of work without substantial financial commitment from funding agencies.

Only one study (Copenhaver et al., 2009) reported using a published adaptation guideline to guide their efforts. This low prevalence may be explained, in part, by the fact that all but one of the existing guidelines (Backer, 2002) had been published in the past 3 years, whereas our sample of studies spans 11 years. Another possible reason is that only two out of the six guidelines (Lee et al., 2008; Smith & Caldwell, 2007) were developed to guide program adaptations for any EBP, whereas the rest provided recommendations for adapting programs that targeted specific conditions, for example, HIV (McKleroy et al., 2006; Wingood & DiClemente, 2008) and substance abuse (Backer, 2002; Kumpfer et al., 2008). However, we would submit that the recommendations present in these guidelines are sufficiently generic that any of them could be employed to adapt programs for a wide variety of disorders. Another possible reason for the rare use of published guidelines is that the guidelines may simply not be feasible for use in time- and resource-limited environments. Finally, those who adapt programs may have difficulty finding the guidelines or simply be unaware of their availability, as the guidelines are not marketed with the original program. Whether use of the guidelines invariably leads to superior products (i.e., better-adapted programs) relative to more informal approaches (e.g., those described in the current report) is a question that should be examined in future research.

Although studies in our sample rarely involved the published guidelines, individual adaptation methods recommended in the six guidelines were frequently employed. More than one third reported conducting literature reviews (this step was recommended by five of the six guidelines) and performed needs assessments (recommended by five). Approximately one half obtained direct feedback about the original program (recommended by two). More than three quarters of the studies evaluated the adapted program to generate additional program revisions (recommended by four guidelines). Nevertheless, of the 36 studies that did not report using an adaptation guideline, none provided information about the methods used to select the individual adaptation approaches employed, such as who decided (e.g., investigators, community advisory board) on the methods to be used to generate suggested modifications to the EBP.

Almost 40% of the articles adhered to the "maintenance of fidelity" standard by explicitly stating that core program components were not modified during the adaptation process. It is possible that a portion of the remaining studies refrained from changing core program elements and simply failed to report this. While the maintenance of fidelity standard appears to be a reasonable criterion, it is important to remember that not all EBPs have undergone steps to identify these core elements. In addition, conducting such appraisals may not be feasible for many groups engaged in adaptation initiatives. In these cases, consulting with the developer of the original program would be an appropriate step to take. Furthermore, none of the studies compared the effectiveness of the adapted and non-adapted programs, and none of the published guidelines recommend a step to compare the effectiveness of the programs. Future studies are necessary to determine whether adapted programs should be evaluated relative to the original and whether the intensity and frequency of the adaptations modify the program's effectiveness.

One of the most important findings of our study is the paucity of information presented in the articles about the methods used to take suggested program adaptations and incorporate them into actual program changes. Of note, none of the published guidelines (Table 4.1) provides recommendations regarding this important step. Only 8% of studies in the sample reported a method for carrying out this phase of the adaptation process. Two studies (Wainberg et al., 2007; Zijlstra et al., 2006) described using a consensus work group–type approach. Wainberg et al. (2007) created an intervention adaptation work group comprising stakeholders and content experts to discuss and adapt program content based on the relevance, cultural appropriateness, and feasibility of the suggested program modifications. Similarly, Zijlstra et al. (2006) convened an expert working group to determine which adaptations to incorporate and provide specific reasons regarding why a suggested adaptation was (or was not) incorporated into the revised program. Explicating the method(s) employed to translate suggested changes into actual programmatic changes is important because different methods likely lead to different program adaptations. Efforts to develop efficient methods for accomplishing this step in the adaptation process are needed. This finding is particularly relevant for T3 translational research efforts that attempt to bridge the gap between research and practice.

The current study also documents that certain types of adaptations occur more commonly than others. A majority of the studies reported making content additions or enhancements during the adaptation process, changing the way certain aspects of the program were delivered, and making cosmetic changes (e.g., changing the name of the program). In contrast, content deletions were reported by less than one fifth of the studies, suggesting that programs undergoing adaptation are far more likely to have elements added than removed. It is possible (and perhaps likely) that the authors of the papers did not report all the adaptations that were made to the various programs. It seems prudent from a reporting standpoint that articles include an exhaustive list of all of their adaptations (presented perhaps as appendices or online), including "accidental" or unplanned adaptations (Galbraith, 2004), and provide the reasons why particular aspects of a program were adapted. This would be useful for others attempting to adapt EBPs for new populations.

Our review has several limitations that warrant consideration. First, our search strategy may have failed to identify all pertinent articles during the search interval (1999–2010). However, we used a broad array of search terms and databases, along with a careful review of the references from all retained articles, in an attempt to eliminate this potential bias. Similarly, our search strategy only identified studies focusing on health, health care, and chronic disease management. It is possible that research on processes and outcomes for program adaptation in other fields, such as education, criminology, and environmental studies, would have yielded different results. However, this review may serve as a model for program adaptation research in other fields.

Much discussion took place among the investigators regarding how to classify the adaptations and adaptation processes employed. In view of this subjectivity, it is possible that a different group of investigators would have classified the items differently, leading to different results. In addition, while a significant majority of the articles provided some description of the adaptation processes used, these descriptions often lacked detail. Our results may therefore not reflect the full range of adaptation methods employed or the types of adaptations actually made.

Full reporting of methods is essential in determining what might constitute an "optimal" approach for adapting EBPs. With better reporting of the individual methods used, we may find that certain approaches are more appropriate for use with different target conditions or populations—for example, certain adaptation steps may be more important in STD prevention programs than for substance abuse treatment programs. In either case, it essential that those who adapt programs be diligent and provide detailed, step-by-step descriptions of their methods. In addition, a detailed report increases its replicability for community agencies and others interested in adapting a program for different audiences. Finally, thorough detailing may help potential program adapters decide whether it is appropriate to use the adapted program directly without making further changes.

This study adds to the limited literature on a very important component of T3 translational research. It provides important information about current program adaptation practices for those seeking to conduct T3 research projects with new settings and populations. Our results demonstrate the use of diverse adaptation approaches and rare use of published guidelines over the past decade. Our study also demonstrates that certain types of adaptations (content additions) occur more frequently than others (content deletions). To advance understanding of how EBPs can be optimally adapted, future research is needed to determine whether systematic approaches in the form of published adaptation guidelines produce superior results relative to current practices.

REFERENCES

Ackermann, R. T., & Marrero, D. G. (2007). Adapting the Diabetes Prevention Program lifestyle intervention for delivery in the community: The YMCA model. *The Diabetes Educator, 33*(1), 69–78. doi:10.1177/0145721706297743

Administration on Aging. (2010). *Evidence-based disease and disability prevention program (EBDDP)*. Retrieved from http://www.aoa.gov/AoARoot/AoA_Programs/HPW/Evidence_Based/index.aspx

Backer, T. E. (2002). *Program fidelity and adaptation in substance abuse prevention, 2002 conference edition*. Washington, DC: Department of Health and Human Services.

Belansky, E. S., Romaniello, C., Morin, C., Uyeki, T., Sawyer, R.L., Scarbro, S., . . . Marshall, J. A. (2006). Adapting and implementing a long-term nutrition and physical activity curriculum to a rural, low-income, biethnic community. *Journal of Nutrition Education and Behavior, 38*, 106–113. doi:10.1016/j.jneb.2005.11.011

Bhana, A., Petersen, I., Mason, A., Mahintsho, Z., Bell, C., & McKay, M. (2004). Children and youth at risk: Adaptation and pilot study of the CHAMP (*Amaqhawe*) programme in South Africa. *African Journal of AIDS Research, 3*(1), 33–41. doi:10.2989/16085900409490316

Burgio, L. D., Collins, I. B., Schmid, B., Wharton, T. W., McCallum, D., & Decoster, J. (2009). Translating the REACH caregiver intervention for use by area agency on aging personnel: The REACH OUT program. *The Gerontologist, 49*(1), 103–116. doi:10.1093/geront/gnp012

Castro, F. G., Barrera, M., & Martinez, C. (2004). The cultural adaptation of prevention interventions: Resolving tensions between fidelity and fit. *Prevention Science, 5*(1), 41–45. doi:10.1023/B:PREV.0000013980.12412.cd

Copenhaver, M., Chowdhury, S., & Altice, F. L. (2009). Adaptation of an evidence-based intervention targeting HIV-infected prisoners transitioning to the community: The process and outcome of formative research for the Positive Living Using Safety (PLUS) intervention. *AIDS Patient Care and STDs, 23*, 277–287. doi:10.1089/apc.2008.0157

Cornelius, J. B., Moneyham, L., & LeGrand, S. (2008). Adaptation of an HIV prevention curriculum for use with older African American women. *Journal of the Association of Nurses in AIDS Care, 19*(1), 16–27. doi:10.1016/j.jana.2007.10.001

D'Angelo, E., Llerena-Ouinn, R., Shapiro, R., Colon, F., Rodriguez, P., Gallagher, K., . . . Beardslee, W. R. (2009). Adaptation of the preventive intervention program for depression for use with predominantly low-income Latino families. *Family Process, 48*, 269–291. doi:10.1111/j.1545-5300.2009.01281.x

Devieux, J. G., Malow, R. M., Jean-Gilles, M. M., Samuels, D., Deschamps, M. M., Ascencio, M. J., . . . Pape, W. J. (2004). Reducing health disparities through culturally sensitive treatment for HIV+ adults in Haiti. *The ABNF Journal: Official Journal of the Association of Black Nursing Faculty In Higher Education, 15*, 109–115.

Diffusion of Effective Behavioral Interventions. (2010). *Diffusion of Effective Behavioral Interventions (DEBI)*. Retrieved from http://www.effectiveinterventions.org/en/AboutDebi/MoreInfo.aspx

Fiscian, V. S., Obeng, E. K., Goldstein, K., Shea, J. A., & Turner, B. J. (2009). Adapting a multifaceted U.S. HIV prevention education program for girls in Ghana. *AIDS Education and Prevention, 21*(1), 67–79. doi:10.1521/aeap.2009.21.1.67

Galbraith, J. (2004). *An examination of the re-invention of a health promotion program: The changes and evolution of "Focus on Kids" HIV prevention program* (Doctoral dissertation). Retrieved from Digital Repository at the University of Maryland (1903/1392).

Galbraith, J., Ricardo, I., Stanton, B., Black, M., Feigelman, S., & Kaljee, L. (1996). Challenges and rewards of involving community in research: An overview of the "Focus on Kids" HIV Risk Reduction Program. *Health Education Quarterly, 23*, 383–394. doi:10.1177/109019819602300308

Gitlin, L. N., Chernett, N. L., Harris, L. F., Palmer, D., Hopkins, P., & Dennis, M. P. (2008). Harvest health: Translation of the chronic disease self-management program for older African Americans in a senior setting. *The Gerontologist, 48* 698–705. doi:10.1093/geront/48.5.698

Hitt, J. C., Robbins, A. S., Galbraith, J. S., Todd, J. D., Patel-Larson, A., McFarlane, J. R., . . . Carey, J. W. (2006). Adaptation and implementation of an evidence-based prevention counseling intervention in Texas. *AIDS Education and Prevention, 18*(4, Suppl. A), 108–118. doi:10.1521/aeap.2006.18.supp.108

Kanowski, L. G., Jorm, A. F., & Hart, L. M. (2009). A mental health first aid training program for Australian Aboriginal and Torres Strait Islander peoples: Description and initial evaluation. *International Journal of Mental Health Systems, 3*(1), 10. doi:10.1186/1752-4458-3-10

Karanja, N., Stevens, V. J., Hollis, J. F., & Kumanyika, S. K. (2002). Steps to soulful living (steps): A weight loss program for African-American women. *Ethnicity & Disease, 12*, 363–371.

Kataoka, S. H., Fuentes, S., O'Donoghue, V. P., Castillo-Campos, P., Bonilla, A., Halsey, K., . . . Wells, K. B. (2006). A community participatory research partnership: The development of a faith-based intervention for children exposed to violence. *Ethnicity & Disease, 16*(1, Suppl. 1), S89–S97.

Komro, K. A., Perry, C. L., Veblen-Mortenson, S., Bosma, L. M., Dudovitz, B. S., Williams, C. L., . . . Toomey, T. L. (2004). Brief report: The adaptation of Project Northland for urban youth. *Journal of Pediatric Psychology, 29*, 457–466. doi:10.1093/jpepsy/jsh049

Kumpfer, K. L., Pinyuchon, M., Teixeira de Melo, A., & Whiteside, H. O. (2008). Cultural adaptation process for international dissemination of the strengthening families program. *Evaluation & the Health Professions, 31*, 226–239. doi:10.1177/0163278708315926

Lee, S. J., Altschul, I., & Mowbray, C. T. (2008). Using planned adaptation to implement evidence-based programs with new populations. *American Journal of Community Psychology, 41*, 290–303. doi:10.1007/s10464-008-9160-5

Lerdboon, P., Pham, V., Green, M., Riel, R., Tho, L. H., Ha, N., . . . Kaljee, L. M. (2008). Strategies for developing gender-specific HIV prevention for adolescents in Vietnam. *AIDS Education and Prevention, 20*, 384–398. doi:10.1521/aeap.2008.20.5.384

Li, X., Wang, B., Fang, X., Zhao, R., Stanton, B., Hong, Y., . . . Yeng, H. (2006). Short-term effect of a cultural adaptation of voluntary counseling and testing among female sex workers in China: A quasi-experimental trial. *AIDS Education and Prevention, 18*, 406–419. doi:10.1521/aeap.2006.18.5.406

Marek, L. I., Brock, D. P., & Sullivan, R. (2006). Cultural adaptations to a family life skills program: Implementation in rural Appalachia. *The Journal of Primary Prevention, 27,* 113–133. doi:10.1007/s10935-005-0017-5

McIntyre, L. L. (2008). Adapting Webster-Stratton's incredible years parent training for children with developmental delay: Findings from a treatment group only study. *Journal of Intellectual Disability Research, 52,* 1176–1192. doi:10.1111/j.1365-2788.2008.01108.x

McKleroy, V. S., Galbraith, J. S., Cummings, B., Jones, P., Harshbarger, C., Collins, C., . . . Carey, J. W. (2006). Adapting evidence-based behavioral interventions for new settings and target populations. *AIDS Education and Prevention, 18(4,* Suppl. A), 59–73. doi:10.1521/aeap.2006.18.supp.59

McTigue, K. M., Conroy, M. B., Hess, R., Bryce, C. L., Fiorillo, A. B., Fischer, G., . . . Simkin-Silverman, L. R. (2009). Using the Internet to translate an evidence-based lifestyle intervention into practice. *Telemedicine and e-Health, 15,* 851–858. doi:10.1089/tmj.2009.0036

Mueller, T. E., Castaneda, C. A., Sainer, S., Martinez, D., Herbst, J. H., Wilkes, A. L., & Villaruel, A. M. (2009). The implementation of a culturally based HIV sexual risk reduction program for Latino youth in a Denver area high school. *AIDS Education and Prevention, 21(5,* Suppl. b), 164–170. doi:10.1521/aeap.2009.21.5_supp.164

National Institute of Mental Health Collaborative HIV/STD Prevention Trial Group. (2007a). The community popular opinion leader HIV programme: Conceptual basis and intervention procedures. *AIDS, 21*(Suppl. 2), S59–S68. doi:10.1097/01.aids.0000266458.49138.fa

National Institute of Mental Health Collaborative HIV/STD Prevention Trial Group. (2007b). Formative study conducted in five countries to adapt the community popular opinion leader intervention. *AIDS, 21*(Suppl. 2), S91–S98. doi:10.1097/01.aids.0000266461.33891.d0

National Institute of Mental Health Collaborative HIV/STD Prevention Trial Group. (2007c). Methodological overview of a five-country community-level HIV/sexually transmitted disease prevention trial. *AIDS, 21*(Suppl. 2), S3–S18. doi:10.1097/01.aids.0000266453.18644.27

Pekmezi, D. W., Neighbors, C. J., Lee, C. S., Gans, K. M., Bock, B. C., Morrow, K. M., & Marcus, B. H. (2009). A culturally adapted physical activity intervention for Latinas: A randomized controlled trial. *American Journal of Preventive Medicine, 37,* 495–500. doi:10.1016/j.amepre.2009.08.023

Punzalan, C., Paxton, K. C., Guentzel, H., Bluthenthal, R. N., Staunton, A. D., Mejia, G., . . . Miranda, J. (2006). Seeking community input to improve implementation of a lifestyle modification program. *Ethnicity & Disease, 16*(1, Suppl. 1), S79–S88.

Quinn, G., Ellison, B. B., Meade, C., Roach, C., Lopez, E., Albrecht, T., & Brandon, T. H. (2006). Adapting smoking relapse-prevention materials for pregnant and postpartum women: Formative research. *Maternal and Child Health Journal, 10,* 235–245. doi:10.1007/s10995-005-0046-y

Reijneveld, S. A., Westhoff, M. H., & Hopman-Rock, M. (2003). Promotion of health and physical activity improves the mental health of elderly immigrants: Results of a group randomised controlled trial among Turkish immigrants in the Netherlands aged 45 and over. *Journal of Epidemiology and Community Health*, *57*, 405–411. doi:10.1136/jech.57.6.405

Rey, G. N., & Sainz, M. T. (2007). Tailoring an intervention model to help indigenous families cope with excessive drinking in Central Mexico. *Salud Mental*, *30*(6), 32–42.

Sarkisian, C. A., Brusuelas, R. J., Steers, W. N., Davidson, M. B., Brown, A. F., Norris, K. C., . . . Mangione, C. M. (2005). Using focus groups of older African Americans and Latinos with diabetes to modify a self-care empowerment intervention. *Ethnicity & Disease*, *15*, 283–291.

Smith, E., & Caldwell, L. (2007). Adapting evidence-based programs to new contexts: What needs to be changed? *The Journal of Rural Health*, *23*(Suppl. 1), 37–41. doi:10.1111/j.1748-0361.2007.00122.x

Social Work Policy Institute. (2010). *Partnerships to promote evidence-based practice*. Retrieved from http://www.socialworkpolicy.org/research/evidence-based-practice-2.html.

Somerville, G. G., Diaz, S., Davis, S., Coleman, K. D., & Taveras, S. (2006). Adapting the popular opinion leader intervention for Latino young migrant men who have sex with men. *AIDS Education and Prevention*, *18*(4, Suppl.), 137–148. doi:10.1521/aeap.2006.18.supp.137

Steiker, L. K. (2008). Making drug and alcohol prevention relevant: Adapting evidence-based curricula to unique adolescent cultures. *Family & Community Health: The Journal of Health Promotion & Maintenance*, *31*(Suppl. 1), S52–S60.

Tsarouk, T., Thompson, E. A., Herting, J. R., Walsh, E., & Randell, B. (2007). Culturally specific adaptation of a prevention intervention: An international collaborative research project. *Addictive Behaviors*, *32*, 1565–1581. doi:10.1016/j.addbeh.2006.11.013

Tsey, K., Whiteside, M., Daly, S., Deemal, A., Gibson, T., Cadet-James, Y., . . . Haswell-Elkins, M. R. (2005). Adapting the "family wellbeing" empowerment program to the needs of remote indigenous school children. *Australian and New Zealand Journal of Public Health*, *29*, 112–116. doi:10.1111/j.1467-842X.2005.tb00059.x

U.S. Department of Health and Human Services. (2010). *SAMHSA's national registry of evidence-based programs and practices*. Retrieved from http://www.nrepp.samhsa.gov/

Villarruel, A. M., Jemmott, L. S., & Jemmott, J. B. (2005). Designing a culturally based intervention to reduce HIV sexual risk for Latino adolescents. *Journal of the Association of Nurses in AIDS Care*, *16*(2), 23–31. doi:10.1016/j.jana.2005.01.001

Wainberg, M. L., McKinnon, K., Mattos, P. E., Pinto, D., Mann, C. G., de Oliveira, C. S., . . . Cournos, F. (2007). A model for adapting evidence-based behavioral interventions to a new culture: HIV prevention for psychiatric patients in Rio de Janeiro, Brazil. *AIDS and Behavior, 11*, 872–883. doi:10.1007/s10461-006-9181-8

Walker, C., Weeks, A., McAvoy, B., & Demetriou, E. (2005). Exploring the role of self-management programmes in caring for people from culturally and linguistically diverse backgrounds in Melbourne, Australia. *Health Expectations, 8*, 315–323. doi:10.1111/j.1369-7625.2005.00343.x

Wegner, L., Flisher, A. J., Caldwell, L. L., Vergnani, T., & Smith, E. A. (2008). Healthwise South Africa: Cultural adaptation of a school-based risk prevention programme. *Health Education Research, 23*, 1085–1096. doi:10.1093/her/cym064

Wingood, G. M., & DiClemente, R. J. (2008). The ADAPT-ITT model: A novel method of adapting evidence-based HIV interventions. *Journal of Acquired Immune Deficiency Syndromes, 47*(Suppl. 1), S40–S46. doi:10.1097/QAI.0b013e3181605df1

Westfall, J. M., Mold, J., & Fagnan, L. (2007). Practice-based research—"Blue Highways" on the NIH Roadmap. *JAMA, 297*, 403–406. doi:10.1001/jama.297.4.403

Woolf, S. H. (2008). The meaning of translational research and why it matters. *JAMA, 299*, 211–213. doi:10.1001/jama.2007.26

Zijlstra, G. A., Tennstedt, S. L., van Haastregt, J. C., van Eijk, J., & Kempen, G. I. (2006). Reducing fear of falling and avoidance of activity in elderly persons: The development of a Dutch version of an American intervention. *Patient Education and Counseling, 62*, 220–227. doi:10.1016/j.pec.2005.07.005

II

FOUR CASE STUDIES FOR TRANSLATING SOCIAL AND BEHAVIORAL SCIENCE TO IMPROVE WELL-BEING, HEALTH, AND PROFESSIONAL PRACTICE

5

PURSUING AND SHARING KNOWLEDGE TO INFORM PRACTICE AND POLICY: THE VALUE OF QUALITATIVE RESEARCH IN TRANSLATIONAL RESEARCH

JEAN M. ISPA

About 15 years ago, for a graduate class in social and emotional development, I assigned an article about links between financial hardship and the quality of young children's home environments. After we had discussed the researchers' methods and the findings, an international student, much puzzled, asked, "Why doesn't your government act on this knowledge?" That I still pause when I remember that question attests to its ongoing, troubling relevance.

As recent appeals for translational research make clear, the responsibility to use sound research findings to inform practice and policy lies with all involved parties—researchers, practitioners, and policymakers (Huston, 2005; National Association for the Education of Young Children & Society for Research in Child Development, 2008; Wethington & Pillemer, 2007).

While writing this chapter, I thought often of how much I have been stimulated by and have learned from the other members of the Early Head Start Research Consortium and the mothers and children who allowed us into their lives. I am also very grateful to the 2009 Bronfenbrenner Conference organizers and volume editors, Elaine Wethington and Rachel Dunifon, for alerting conference participants to important references and for providing me with invaluable suggestions for elaboration and clarification of points made in my original conference paper. I also want to thank my daughter, Simone Ispa-Landa, and my graduate research assistant, J. Claire Cook, for very constructive feedback on earlier drafts.

As a researcher and professor, I think that there are two general ways in which academics can positively influence policy and practice. First, we should pursue knowledge about the effects of various environmental conditions on the current and long-term functioning of individuals and families. This goal requires that we listen to practitioners, policymakers, and service recipients, as well as to other researchers, and that we offer to submit their promising ideas to the scrutiny of evaluation research. Second, we have the obligation to share what we know with policymakers, practitioners, and the public.

In this chapter, I reflect on my experiences in conducting and sharing translational research. I focus particularly on the circumstances that led me to adopt qualitative methods and the challenges and satisfactions that have followed. To prepare for the 2009 Bronfenbrenner Conference, I read articles promoting translational research and reporting on best practices. The publications I came across (e.g., Huston, 2005; Maccoby, Kahn, & Everett, 1983; McCall, 2009; National Association for the Education of Young Children & Society for Research in Child Development, 2008; Wethington & Pillemer, 2007) were inspiring and helped me to clarify and expand my thoughts. I noticed, however, that most of the pieces I was reading emphasized the construction and uses of large data sets amenable to sophisticated statistical analyses. I am a proponent of such research and have engaged in it myself as an eager participant in the Early Head Start Research Consortium, which has been evaluating the short- and long-term effects of Early Head Start on a large, nationwide sample of children and parents (original $n = 3,001$) for the past 15 years. However, I would also like to tout the value of small-scale qualitative research for translational research purposes.

In this chapter, I first tell how I was introduced to qualitative research. Because most of these experiences have occurred in the context of my involvement in Early Head Start–related research, I provide some background on the establishment of Early Head Start and the research consortium charged with its evaluation. Next, in the section Pursuing Knowledge—Why We Decided to Use Qualitative Methods, I describe the circumstances that led me and my colleagues to adopt qualitative research approaches. In Gearing Up, I recall how I learned qualitative research strategies. Then, in the section Strengths of Qualitative and Mixed Method Approaches, I use examples from specific studies to explain the strengths of qualitative and mixed methods approaches for advancing and sharing knowledge. The section Sharing Knowledge focuses on the readability of case studies and other qualitative works. Accessibility to lay audiences is a potential key benefit of qualitative reporting. In the final section, Dilemmas, I reflect on the journey that I have experienced in my work as a qualitative researcher. Here I share some of the major challenges and high points that have come my way.

ESTABLISHMENT OF EARLY HEAD START AND THE EARLY HEAD START RESEARCH CONSORTIUM

Early Head Start was inaugurated in 1995 to provide child development and family support services to low-income parents and children from the time of pregnancy until children reach the age of 3. Its overarching goal is to close the achievement gap between children living in poverty and more advantaged children by improving prenatal health and emotional, social, cognitive, and physical development during infancy and toddlerhood. Programs may choose to follow one of three models: home-visiting, center-based, or mixed. The mixed model allows families to choose home-visiting or center-based care, depending on their personal needs. All models employ a two-generational approach, focusing not only on the direct needs of children for growth-promoting physical, emotional, and educational care but also on the needs of parents (for assistance in obtaining housing, education, employment, mental health services, etc.). Two-generational programs rest on the belief that services that benefit parents indirectly benefit children.

Congress first allocated funding for Early Head Start in 1994 after being convinced by two lines of research that pointed to the importance of support for children in low-income families as soon after conception as possible. One of these lines of research concerned brain development. It provided evidence of the malleability (and vulnerability) of the brain during the prenatal and infant–toddler periods. It had become clear that during these initial stages of life, nutrition, stress, caregiver responsivity, and age-appropriate stimulation have significant near- and long-term consequences for the developing brain (Shonkoff & Phillips, 2000).

The second influential line of research concerned the school success of graduates of Head Start. Head Start had been established in 1965 to provide comprehensive health and early childhood education services to 3- and 4-year-olds from impoverished families. The results of evaluations had been mixed. Large-scale studies had indicated that at entrance to kindergarten, children who had attended Head Start were more ready for school than were their counterparts who had not participated in the program. Unfortunately, however, their advantage appeared to have faded out by third grade. (See Zigler & Muenchow, 1992, for an excellent overview and critique of then-available Head Start evaluations.) Together, these two lines of research fueled concerns that for children living in poverty, interventions starting at age 3 or 4 begin too late.

Immediately after Congress authorized the establishment of Early Head Start, the Secretary of the Department of Health and Human Services appointed the Advisory Committee on Services for Families with Infants and Toddlers and asked members to create a blueprint for the program. One of the group's recommendations was to include a strong research component for the purposes of program evaluation and continuous improvement (Administration on Children, Youth and Families, 1994). Congress agreed. The resultant request for proposals (RFP) called for a national consortium of researchers who would participate in the evaluation of 17 of the initial 68 Early Head Start sites scattered across the country.

One of the criticisms of the early evaluations of Head Start, such as the Westinghouse–Ohio study (Cicirelli, 1969), was that the researchers had compared Head Start graduates with a comparison group chosen retrospectively, after the children had begun attending public school. There was thus no way to be sure that the Head Start and comparison children did not differ on key variables even before some of the children began attending Head Start. Moreover, the first evaluations relied on IQ scores as their outcome measures even though it was known that IQ tests do not validly assess minority and low-income children's potential to achieve. Especially because this conference honors Urie Bronfenbrenner's legacy, it is worth noting that when the first Head Start evaluations were being designed, he, Edward Zigler, and Edmund Gordon strongly argued with officials in the evaluation division of the Office of Economic Opportunity against these suspect approaches, but to no avail (Zigler & Muenchow, 1992). The RFP calling for the national evaluation of Early Head Start reflected its designers' recognition of these problems. The evaluation was to be based on a random assignment design. In other words, applicants would be randomly assigned to either receive Early Head Start services or to participate in the evaluation only as members of the comparison group.

Mathematica Policy Research, Inc., and Columbia University's Center for Children and Families won the contracts to coordinate the national evaluation with researchers from 15 universities. Funding continued for 5 years, allowing longitudinal data to be collected on families entering the study during 3 consecutive years (1996, 1997, and 1998). Assessments were conducted not just via standardized tests of intelligence but also on children's social, emotional, cognitive, language, and physical development; the emotional and learning climate of their home environments; and their parents' attitudes, child rearing behaviors, physical and mental health, and progress toward self-sufficiency. These assessments took place when children were 14, 24, and 36 months old. In addition, parents were interviewed about their needs, resources, and service usage 6, 15, and 26 months after random assignment and when children exited the program at age 3. Finally, program implementation level was assessed during three site visits.

The RFP also had a second prong that was unique in that it promised additional funding over the same 5 years for separate "local" research focusing on the families, the staff, and the program at individual research sites. It was hoped that local research would complement the national evaluation by adding in-depth knowledge informed by sensitivity to community context. Researchers, program directors, and staff were to form a partnership with the goal that researchers and practitioners would benefit each other. Practitioners would be encouraged to suggest research ideas and provide access to data, and researchers would in turn provide practitioners with research-based information that they could use for program improvement purposes. Years later, I found out that Urie Bronfenbrenner gave the Advisory Committee and the RFP writers the idea for this dual-funding approach.

Funding of the program's evaluation has extended far beyond the initial 3-year plan. So far, data have also been collected when children were approaching kindergarten age and, most recently, when they were in fifth grade. At present, plans are under way to reconnect with families to obtain current addresses and other contact information so that we can locate them should funding become available when children are of high school age.

The evaluation results have provided support for the effectiveness of the program. At age 3, children who had been in Early Head Start scored modestly better on a wide range of socioemotional and cognitive measures than did children who were in the comparison group. Concomitantly, program group parents demonstrated more positive child rearing behaviors than did parents in the comparison group. Not surprisingly, families in well-implemented programs and families that enrolled during pregnancy showed the strongest benefits. Other subgroups with particularly strong benefits included African American families and families with a moderate number of demographic risk factors (Administration for Children and Families, 2002a). The program group advantage was still evident when children were about to enter kindergarten (Administration for Children and Families, 2006) but had decreased by fifth grade as children in both groups encountered similar schooling and neighborhood environments.

The positive results (especially promising because they were based on data collected when Early Head Start was barely off the ground) have been credited as responsible for lawmakers' willingness to fund its expansion. The evaluation has thus been important not only because it generated evidence-based ideas for program improvement but also because of the confidence it has generated in politicians whose votes determine its very existence.

PURSUING KNOWLEDGE: WHY WE DECIDED TO USE QUALITATIVE METHODS

Soon after learning that we had been awarded one of the grants allowing us to participate in the national evaluation and focus on a specific program, Kathy Thornburg, Mark Fine, and I scheduled our first meeting with our site's director. At this point we knew little about her plans except that she wanted to employ a home-visiting model for her program. The meeting was at a McDonald's along the highway, at the halfway mark between our university offices and the building where she was working to establish the new program. It was a location that required each party to drive an equal distance. Looking back, I think of the decision to meet there as symbolic of the commitment on both sides to make this a two-way partnership.

In that spirit, at that first meeting, we asked the director to share with us her pressing concerns and to tell us what she would like us to learn through the course of the research study. To my surprise and, I must admit, my consternation, she told us that she would like us to help her and her staff of home visitors understand more about the mothers and children they would soon be recruiting—how they live, what they think and feel about their relationships, and what they see as their needs. She expected (correctly) that most of the mothers and infants her particular Early Head Start program would serve would be African American, and the great majority of the mothers would be very young, single, and still living with their own mothers. She was worried that home visitors had little understanding of this population of families. Some had social work backgrounds and knew how to access social services for clients, but they had little background regarding child development or family dynamics. Most had had little or no direct contact with impoverished teen mothers. She thought that the more they knew about the personal lives of the young mothers, children, and families they were about to serve, the more determined they would be to help them and the more effectively they would communicate with them.

One of my colleagues asked her if she would prefer that we use qualitative or quantitative methods. She was quite definite that the study should be qualitative because she wanted rich descriptions of as many aspects of the families' lives as we could access, and she wanted opportunities for the families and her staff to share unexpected perspectives. She hoped that a qualitative study would shed light on the inner workings of the families her staff would be trying to support and that it would lend itself to writings that included quotations and case studies whose points would be accessible to lay audiences.

This was a tall order for us. The three of us had been schooled in quantitative methods and knew little about qualitative methods. Moreover, we had had little experience in conducting research with African American low-income families. Nevertheless, we nodded that this was what we would do. Why did we agree to the director's request? One reason was that we, too, were curious about the lives of the families the program would be serving. We saw our (and the field's) limited knowledge of this population as a serious gap that needed to be addressed. The second reason was pragmatic. We knew that the director's long-term commitment to our research endeavor, however it might shape up, was essential, and we wanted to start out making a positive impression on her. (See Green, Mulvey, Fisher, and Rudacille, 1996, for additional examples of the accommodations both sides must make to support program–researcher partnerships.)

On the drive back from this first meeting, we decided that we would learn about qualitative methods and that we would each set out to get to know three Early Head Start families through multiple interviews with mothers in the program, relatives and friends close to them, and their home visitors. The initial plan was to interview each of nine mothers and her family members three times a year for 5 years, and the home visitors and other staff once a year. In actuality, our data were so compelling that 5 years after what was to have been the end of the project, we requested (and received) funding to return to conduct follow-up interviews with the children (now 10 and 11 years old) and their parents. A book, *Keepin' On: The Everyday Struggles of Young Families in Poverty* (Ispa, Thornburg, & Fine, 2006), and several articles (Brookes, Summers, Thornburg, Ispa, & Lane, 2006; Ispa & Halgunseth, 2004; Sharp & Ispa, 2009) describe our qualitative findings pertaining to the program and to the mothers' thoughts and experiences relative to multiple levels of their ecological systems.

Over the years, we used a variety of methods to collect data for our local project. Because we wanted to keep the door open for mixed method approaches, we relied on a few instruments developed for quantitative analysis. Our main focus, however, followed our commitment to the director's request and involved the collection and analysis of qualitative data.

GEARING UP

Our "transformation" into qualitative as well as quantitative researchers was exciting but not smooth. Following colleagues' recommendations, we read articles on feminist theory (e.g., Collins, 1990; Thompson, 1992; Wuest, 1995) to think more about our responsibility to convey the complexities of the day-to-day lives of the marginalized, understudied people we were getting to know. We read books such as Patton's (1990) and Strauss and Corbin's (1998) texts on qualitative methods. A research assistant taking a course on qualitative methods knew that I was searching for guidance. She showed me the syllabus and suggested that I read two books the professor had recommended as excellent examples of the products of qualitative investigation: *Slim's Table: Race, Respectability, and Masculinity* (Duneier, 1992) and *Number Our Days* (Myerhoff, 1978). These works greatly increased my appreciation for the purposes and end results of qualitative research; still, I struggled to understand how to actually do it. How would I conduct interviews in the constantly alert manner demanded by this type of research, and how would I simultaneously keep my eyes open to take in the larger contexts of the families' surroundings? When one distributes questionnaires or conducts interviews that will be analyzed quantitatively, it is often important that all respondents be asked the same questions in the same order and in the same way. While the qualitative interviewer also seeks to ask certain questions, the order and wording are less predetermined, and there is license to pursue unplanned leads in respondents' comments and gestures. Especially for the novice interviewer, this license can feel like a burden, an enormous demand for sensitivity and quick-mindedness.

I was helped by tips shared in books such as those by Kvale (1996) and Rubin and Rubin (1995) on qualitative interviewing techniques. In these books, I read about the importance of wording choices, active listening, and ways to balance plans for the direction of interviews with flexibility to mean-der when something else is weighing on interviewees' minds. I also benefited from postinterview discussions with my graduate research assistant, Elizabeth Sharp. During these discussions, many of which occurred on our long drives back home, we honestly reflected on strategies that had gone well and those that had not. For example, early on we wondered whether one mother in particular would be more open with us if we did not have our sheets of paper with our interview questions with us. Before the next visit, we rehearsed the questions several times, then left the sheets of paper in the car. The interview this time generated much richer dialogue and a warmer atmosphere than the one before. In hindsight, this lesson seems elementary. I share it because it illustrates the place at which we started, the value of flexibility, and the self-reflection and perspective taking that had to occur.

Consultations with experienced qualitative researchers were also of great importance. During the first 2 years of the project, we invited Carol McAllister, a member of the Early Head Start Research Consortium, and later Gina Barclay-McLaughlin, a consultant to the consortium, to visit us in Columbia and hold workshops for our team. They tutored us regarding the establishment of relationships with research participants and the importance of looking for the meanings that participants gave to the events in their lives. I remember one day in particular. At the time, I was worried not so much about the amount of data facing us (eventually it would be over 2,000 typed pages of transcripts and field notes) as about my ability to detect key themes in the families' lives. Barclay-McLaughlin read a few of our transcripts and discussed with us some of the salient themes that seemed to be emerging. During the subsequent years, our team continued to meet regularly to share and debate sources and inter-pretations. Because our work was longitudinal, over the years of the study the frequent recurrence of certain comments and observations captured our atten-tion and facilitated our identification of central patterns.

I must also give credit to QSR NVivo, the software package that we used to manage, data and to the accompanying manuals. NVivo, like other software programs developed to help researchers manage and manipulate qualitative data, cannot do the conceptual work of identifying themes, but it is invaluable as an organizational aid when large amounts of text and other materials must be analyzed. I especially benefited from a book by Bazeley and Richards (2000) that guides readers through the multiple steps of qualitative analysis, from initial coding to identification of themes and their interrelationships.

STRENGTHS OF QUALITATIVE AND MIXED METHOD APPROACHES

It is often said that qualitative methods allow researchers to give a voice to those whom society marginalizes and that they permit the generation of rich data about circumstances and processes that we know too little about to devise revealing Likert-type items or other assessments (Merrick, 1999; Moffitt, 2000). Qualitative methods can unearth and explore unknown or poorly understood patterns and processes. Though qualitatively derived findings cannot be assumed to be generalizable, they can lead to hypotheses that can be tested using quantitative methods and to effective wording of questionnaire and interview items (Creswell, 1998; Moffitt, 2000). A related point is that qualitative methods can elicit nuanced data that help to explain or qualify the processes thought to lead to quantitative findings (Huston, 2005; McCall, 2009).

An example from our research concerns the findings of the Early Head Start national evaluation showing that mothers in the program were more likely to read to their children than mothers in the comparison group (Love et al., 2005). Our qualitative analyses suggested one unexpected mechanism explaining how this occurred in some families. Having been told by home visitors (a) that it is important to read to infants and toddlers and (b) that children thrive when their parents are responsive to reasonable requests, some mothers in the program seemed more willing than they otherwise would have been to respond positively to toddlers' requests to be read to. In other words, the path to increased book reading was not just from program messages about the importance of reading to increased maternal book-reading rates. It was also through toddler initiation.

The distinction is important from both a researcher and a practitioner standpoint. For researchers, it signals the importance of investigating reciprocal influences between parental book-reading and toddler characteristics, not just one-way, parent-to-child influences. This transactional view was exemplified in a quantitative study using the entire Early Head Start sample to examine maternal book-reading. Raikes et al. (2006) found that mothers' frequency of reading to their 2-year-olds was predicted by toddlers' vocabulary development a year earlier.

For practitioners, consideration of reciprocal effects opens up the possibility of an additional strategy to increase parental reading to children. Besides talking directly with parents about the importance of reading to children and explaining age-appropriate reading strategies, our observation suggests that it would be helpful to make efforts to facilitate children's interest in being read to, even if that means seeing to it that enjoyable reading experiences occur outside the home, in child care settings, or during home visits. If our hypothesis is correct, such experiences will heighten the likelihood that children will ask parents to also read to them, initiating a snowball effect wherein parents agree to do so, children are reinforced to ask again, and the cycle gathers momentum until enjoyable book-reading times are established in the home.

An article I wrote with a graduate research assistant (Ispa & Halgunseth, 2004) provides another illustration of the potential for symbiosis between qualitative research and quantitatively derived findings. Earlier quantitative studies had found higher frequencies of physical punishment by African American parents than by White parents of similar socioeconomic status (e.g., Giles-Sims, Straus, & Sugarman, 1995). We thought we might be able to shed light on the reasons for the high frequencies among low-income African American mothers if we scoured our transcripts for comments about discipline. In so doing, we detected telling themes. Repeated comments indicated that mothers believed that physical punishment is necessary because even very young children "know better," and unchecked early misbehavior portends very big problems when children reach adolescence. Mothers' mental construction of good parenting seemed to involve high levels of vigilance and strictness lest children grow up defiant and succumb to "the streets." One mother expressed the sentiments of the others when she explained that for African American children growing up in the context of racism and poverty, there is "no room for error." We also noticed that our sample of African American parents used different terms for physical punishment depending on its severity and the body part struck. That observation led to our recommendation that questionnaire items for use in quantitative studies be worded in accordance with the terminology in use by the target population. It also led to a recommendation addressed to practitioners that they be careful about wording. One can imagine a parent educator telling a group of parents that they should not spank their children, and the parents thinking that they do not *spank* their children, but merely *pop* them.

Another advantage of qualitative methods as a complement to large-scale evaluations is that they are suited to the discovery of local factors that influence program implementation and program effects in important ways.

Qualitative research can dig beneath statements about program standards to document problems and adjustments that were made in response to local conditions (including characteristics of the program staff, the clientele, and the community).

Two examples come immediately to mind. The Early Head Start site with which I was affiliated served mostly young single mothers and their children. Because many of the mothers were still living with their own mothers, over time the staff realized that they could not make much headway changing the child rearing practices to which toddlers were exposed unless they also involved the children's grandmothers. Some staff followed up on this realization by trying to adjust parent education activities and messages to take both generations into account. Home-visiting times were changed to accommodate the schedules of grandmothers as well as mothers; both generations were invited to evening and weekend meetings at the Early Head Start center. Efforts were made to draw the grandparents into conversations about their reservations concerning the child rearing strategies the home visitors were working to encourage.

Another challenge arrived as welfare reform came into play. Because single mothers were now required to work, home visitors had to make adjustments in their visiting times, and for some this became a major obstacle because they either were afraid or simply did not want to enter mothers' neighborhoods at night or on weekends. Especially during the first 2 years of our study, before major staffing changes occurred, we heard from mothers about their disappointment over broken and simply not-scheduled appointments. Explanations surfaced during our interviews with home visitors, who told us of their unwillingness to work irregular hours, their fears concerning the mothers' neighborhoods, and, unfortunately, in the case of two, their general disapproval of unmarried teen mothers (Brookes, Summers, et al., 2006; Brookes, Thornburg, & Ispa, 2006). Because it is impossible to anticipate or control for all aspects of a community or historical events that affect a program and its clients, a preplanned evaluation with standard items cannot be expected to capture all relevant variables.

Elizabeth Sharp and I also used a qualitative approach to try to shed some light on the national evaluation finding that at age 2, boys seemed to benefit more from Early Head Start than girls (Administration for Children and Families, 2002b). Because our local sample was almost entirely African American, we reviewed the literature specifically on gender socialization in low-income African American families and then analyzed mothers' gender-related comments from the time when we first met them to the time when children were 10 or 11. The extant literature portrayed mothers as holding essentialist beliefs that "boys will be boys" and that girls are more capable than boys of growing up to be independent and strong (e.g., Hill &

Zimmerman, 1995; Wood, Kaplan, & McLoyd, 2007). However, these studies almost all sampled mothers of adolescents; adolescents' behavior might have influenced mothers' thoughts. Our data permitted us to examine mothers' beliefs and goals much earlier. The result was a qualitative study (Sharp & Ispa, 2009) suggesting that long before children reached adolescence, mothers' goals for daughters centered on independence and strength, whereas goals for sons focused on hopes that they would grow up to be different from their fathers—that is, responsible and kind to women. We also saw that these goals were clouded by fatalism founded in mothers' negative personal experiences. In line with feminist theory that gender is constructed and therefore alterable, we recommended that courses and in-service trainings for social service providers teach critical appraisal of gendered discourse to facilitate self-reflection and willingness to counter negative images that are likely communicated to children. It will be important to learn whether the slightly higher benefit to boys is replicated in studies of other early intervention programs and, if so, whether it is due to staff's ability to counter negative expectations about boys' futures.

At present, I am working on a qualitative study whose inspiration is drawn from the results of quantitative analyses indicating that maternal intrusiveness is more likely to predict toddler negativity and poor mother–toddler relationship quality in European American families than in African American or Mexican American families (Ispa et al., 2004). Some speculate that intrusiveness may be more likely to occur in the context of warmth in some ethnic groups than in others. However, the global rating systems used to code observational data typically make it impossible to test this hypothesis. Global ratings cannot be used to determine whether children tend to receive certain types of intrusiveness more calmly than other types or whether the buffering effects of maternal warmth are associated with warmth displayed generally or specifically during intrusive acts. My graduate students and I have coded in detail the interfering behaviors of 28 mothers, the affect accompanying those behaviors, and the reactions of their children to each interruption of self-initiated play. In future quantitative analyses based on larger samples and across ethnic groups, we plan to examine interconnections among the interfering behaviors we have identified and their relations to child outcomes.

Deeper understanding of the quality and consequences of parental intrusiveness is important in an increasingly diverse society. Parent educators employed by programs like Early Head Start typically value the autonomy-granting parenting behaviors that tend to be valued and effective in middle class European American families. Research unraveling intrusiveness has the potential to help social service professionals become more respectful of cultural diversity in parenting patterns. It may also lead to distinctions between intrusive behaviors that are benign, or even beneficial, and those that have negative implications in particular cultural groups.

The examples above focus on showing how qualitative findings can illuminate the mechanisms behind quantitative findings. In the reverse process, investigators use hypotheses derived from qualitative studies to drive research using quantitative methods to determine whether those ideas are generalizable. A case in point is a study that grew out of our qualitatively derived impression that mothers' personality is a factor in the quality of the relationship that develops between them and the home visitors. We administered personality and working alliance measures to mothers and home visitors and collected records on time spent in home visits. Statistical analyses using hierarchical linear modeling revealed that mothers' negative emotionality (the tendency to experience negative moods, depression, anger, or anxiety) predicted both higher relationship satisfaction and more time spent in home visits (Sharp, Ispa, Thornburg, & Lane, 2003). This finding provides food for thought in that it suggests that home visitors should be aware of the disproportionate pull they may feel from mothers who are prone to negative emotions.

SHARING KNOWLEDGE

Another reason to conduct qualitative research—a reason that has moved me very much—is that it is well suited to the generation of writing that is interesting and accessible to lay audiences. In a recent article on translational research, McCall (2009) commented that knowledge from research tends to be conveyed in "small, isolated, and disjointed pieces" (p. 8) that practitioners and policymakers find difficult to grasp and use. Case studies and other forms of reporting of qualitative work have the potential to weave discrete findings, and the theories behind them, together to create holistic portrayals of individuals, groups, programs, and communities. What is more, these accounts can be written in language that is accessible and interesting to general audiences.

I have felt gratified by readers' comments that a case study I wrote following painstaking analysis reads like a novel, or that an article based on qualitative analysis of observations and interviews in a Russian child care center (Ispa, 2002) was "fun to read." The pieces kept readers' attention, thereby allowing me to get some key points across. I believe that it will make a difference if people, including those who have not been schooled in reading academic papers or the results of statistical tests, gain some insight into the lives of people unlike themselves. I want them to recognize that in many ways the thoughts, joys, and struggles of those others are similar to their own, and I want them to understand the reasons for some of the behavior patterns that they look askance at. I am hoping that, as a consequence, they will adopt more sympathetic attitudes, treat people with more dignity, and advocate for policies, programs, and practices that have the potential to help people like those I have portrayed.

In my college sophomore year, I took a large introductory course in human development. Urie Bronfenbrenner was the professor. It was in that class that I learned the distinction between *necessary* and *sufficient*. It was a principle that was important to Bronfenbrenner; I remember that he kept coming back to it in his lectures. To my mind, quantitative methods are necessary, but not sufficient, and the same is true of qualitative methods. Interpretation of national evaluation results is likely to be much enhanced when both approaches are applied. The examples above are illustrative.

Large-scale survey methods and global ratings followed by complex statistical tests with numerous controls were essential to determine Early Head Start impacts, ethnic group differences, and the generalizability of relations between certain child rearing practices and their predictors and outcomes. Qualitative research cannot speak to the generalizability of the themes it uncovers, however compelling they may seem to the researchers. Follow-up statistical analyses on data from new, much larger samples are necessary to test the validity and generalizability of those themes. Furthermore, one must recognize that qualitative data gathered from interviews are inevitably colored by the perceptions of one's interviewees. This, in fact, is what one seeks in qualitative investigations; one wants to know how people think about certain issues, what meanings they have given to the events in their lives. As one develops respect and fondness for participants, it is then all too easy to forget that they may attribute causation where there is none, misinterpret the motivations of others, and not acknowledge (even to themselves) some of the forces that drive their decisions and actions. This means that the qualitative researcher must maintain a certain vigilance, striving to understand the viewpoints of participants while also maintaining a respectful, guarded intellectual distance that prioritizes critical analysis.

Qualitative methods have allowed us to delve deeply into our small sample of African American mothers' beliefs and behaviors, connect them to contextual factors, and write case studies that speak to lay as well as professional audiences. Future studies using quantitative methods will inform us of the prevalence of the parental behaviors and ideas we have identified and their links to child outcomes and parental openness to change. Practice and policy can be well served by investigations that draw on the strengths of both qualitative and quantitative approaches.

DILEMMAS

Our charge for the 2009 Bronfenbrenner Conference was to share some of the issues we have encountered as we have proceeded with our work. I will focus on a few that seem specific to the conduct of qualitative research.

As I have thought about the dilemmas my team and I have faced, I have realized that they fall into two sets—dilemmas occasioned when researchers learn of problems and feel ethically obliged to help, and dilemmas occasioned as one tries to manage researcher–participant relationships that border on, but cannot really become, friendships. For examples, I draw on my experiences conducting research involving Early Head Start families because the frequency with which we talked to mothers and the nature of the questions we posed gave prominence to both sets of issues. I end with a third set of issues, those involving career advancement barriers for qualitative researchers.

Dilemmas Occasioned When Researchers Learn of Problems and Feel Ethically Obliged to Help

I wholeheartedly agree with McCall (2009) that programs should not be evaluated in their first year; it may take several cohorts of clients before staff members have learned how to implement a program with fidelity to their preferred model. However, the Early Head Start program that we were charged to evaluate was in its first year when the national evaluation began. As mentioned earlier, in the course of our early interviews with the local site director, home visitors, and mothers, it became evident that there were serious problems in the delivery of our local Early Head Start program. These problems were in part due to gaps in home-visitor knowledge about infant and toddler development and, in several cases, sadly, to a poor work ethic and negative attitudes about adolescent pregnancy. Some home visitors did not reserve time for teaching about child development, instead focusing almost all of their efforts on helping mothers access various social services. A related problem was the tendency of some home visitors to attend to families in crisis at the expense of families whose needs seemed less urgent. We also noted two boundary issues. Even the most skilled home visitors sometimes found it difficult to negotiate the line between professional and friend in their relationships with mothers. In addition, in a couple of cases, home visitors ran the risk of enabling mothers to become dependent on them. We worried that mothers in these relationships would have a hard time separating from home visitors after their children aged out of the program.

An objective-outsider stance would have required us to record our observations and walk away. We would not have wanted to sacrifice the integrity of the research design by intervening in the program's and families' behalf. That is not what happened, however. Part of the reason was structural; as mentioned above, in joining the Early Head Start Research Consortium, we had agreed to create a university–program partnership in which research would be used to inform the program itself. Recall that continuous program improvement was mandated in the legislation that established Early Head

Start. Because of the service delivery problems we saw during the first year of the program, we offered to add the provision of educational activities to our set of responsibilities—a role in line with the notion of a partnership but alien to the notion of disinterested researcher. The director was glad to have our help. We were now obliged not only to take note of program problems but also to try to help rectify them.

In this role, we engaged in two activities. One involved sharing some quantitative data with the administrators and home visitors. Much of these data were demographic (e.g., maternal educational level, age, marital status, income averages and ranges), but some were more psychological, such as average scores and ranges on measures of maternal depression, vocabulary knowledge, and knowledge of infant development. We hoped these data would help staff by giving them a picture of some key characteristics of the families they were serving.

The other activity was more elaborate and more clearly of an interventionist nature. After discovering that the home visitors had had almost no prior coursework on infant and toddler development or on principles of family interaction, we offered to provide a series of workshops on these topics. The director enthusiastically agreed and required her staff to attend. We and our graduate students led multiple in-service trainings during the first 2 years of our affiliation with the program. We did not study the effectiveness of these efforts in terms of improved home-visitor knowledge or service to families. In the future, it would behoove evaluators to determine the usefulness of models wherein researchers assume teacher as well as evaluator roles.

We were also faced with serious dilemmas as we learned about the many problems of individual families participating in our case study research. Should we give advice to mothers, or give them referrals, when we thought such was necessary? Should we give them a few dollars when we saw desperate need? One situation stands out as particularly troubling at the time. It occurred in the third or fourth year of our study. By now there was mutual affection and trust between me and this mother. I knew she loved her children dearly and did everything she could for them. I also knew that she used corporal punishment, but what I had witnessed during prior visits had not alarmed me. I am not a proponent of corporal punishment, but I was familiar with the research literature suggesting that it is not damaging when used in the context of warm, loving relationships (Deater-Deckard & Dodge, 1997). I also knew that this mother's home visitor was working with her on other ways to discipline her children and that she was receptive to these messages. On this day, however, before my eyes and those of my graduate assistant, she spanked her son with more force than was acceptable. The graduate student had never been to this home before and thus had no prior relationship with the family. The next day, she came to my office to insist that we call the Division of Family Services to report child abuse.

I thought this was the wrong thing to do. I thought such a call had the clear potential to do much more harm than good. I knew a lot about the strengths of this mother, and I knew that the children, as well as the mother, would be devastated should they be taken from her. I admit that I was also troubled by a lesser, selfish, concern: I knew it would end the mother's willingness to have me in her home, which would certainly be a problem for our longitudinal study. Luckily, there was an alternative to doing nothing or calling the hotline. I called her home visitor, who completely agreed that "the authorities" should not be brought in and that instead she should increase her attention to this mother's parenting education needs.

This is but one extreme example of dilemmas we faced that involved not only ethical considerations but also potential insults to the integrity of our research. There were instances when one of us gave child rearing advice or gave mothers telephone numbers to call for additional help. I am not saying that we always made the right decisions—I am just noting that ethical issues beset qualitative researchers fairly often.

In fact, looking back, I think the types of dilemmas we encountered as we grappled with decisions about whether, when, and how to intervene are inevitable when one conducts qualitative research with at-risk families and with programs that serve them. For one, the relationships we developed with staff and families during many long interviews for our qualitative project allowed us to learn more about individual lives than I think we would ever have learned had we restricted ourselves to the collection of quantitative data. In addition, the qualitative researcher is less concerned than his or her quantitative counterpart about maintaining neutrality. Qualitative researchers accept the fact that something about them or something they did probably influenced their participants, even if just momentarily. It is then their responsibility to share, in their research reports, features of themselves that may have affected the content or quality of the data they obtained (Merrick, 1999; Richards & Morse, 2007).

Challenges in Managing Imbalanced Relationships:
Impression Management and Role Ambiguity

Another set of issues involves the nature of the researcher–participant relationship, especially when the researcher has elicited private information and there is a clear imbalance in the socioeconomic statuses of the two. These issues include questions about where and how to draw the line between researcher and friend and how to manage one's identity. I know that service providers face these dilemmas also (Brookes, Thornburg, & Ispa, 2006; Musick & Stott, 2000).

As indicated above, our interview questions during visits with the mothers in our Early Head Start case study project elicited some personal information. As time went on and we learned the individual proclivities of each participant, we learned how best to make each one feel comfortable sharing her private thoughts with us. Mothers, fathers, grandmothers, and home visitors told us about their joys and heartaches, their hopes, successes, and failures. Mothers complained about people close to them and about their living, schooling, and work situations. Sometimes they complained about their Early Head Start home visitors. Qualitative research, especially if it is longitudinal, involving repeated interactions, has great potential to precipitate feelings of closeness between investigator and research participant. In many cases, it does not afford the interpersonal distance that is built into the data collector–participant relationship typical of quantitative research designs. Nonetheless, after each interview, we left town and usually did not call back for weeks. I often felt bad about this. Had my research participants been my usual-life friends, I surely would have called back the day after they had confided upsetting emotions and thoughts. Instead, returning to home and campus, I immediately became immersed in my family life (I still had two sons at home) and the mountains of work that always awaited me. I recall times when mothers asked why I had disappeared for so long. It is still a little painful to think about, and I do not have a good solution.

Finally, and relatedly, there are identity presentation dilemmas. The qualitative researcher wants to maximize the participant's comfort in his or her presence and thereby the amount of information that is revealed. How much, then, should she tell about herself? Participants in my research knew that I am employed by the University of Missouri and that I am married and have three children. Unlike my friends, they knew little about the quality of my relationships in these important aspects of my life. Disclosures tended to be one way, by design.

One example comes especially to mind because it involves my decision to hide a simple fact about myself—my age. I was 49 when I met Andreya, a young mother about whom I later wrote a detailed case study (Ispa & Sharp, 2006). She was 19 and had a 1-year-old son. When, at our first meeting, I asked her about her family members, she volunteered that her mother was 35 and her grandmother was 64. Her voice conveyed a sense that 64 is *very* old. I was momentarily taken aback. I was already 14 years older than her son's grandmother, yet not even close to being one myself, and I was only 15 years younger than her son's *great*-grandmother. The differences in our roles at the given ages starkly captured the socioeconomic and life course differences between me and the members of this family. I resolved never to let them know my age because I feared it would put too much distance between us. Perhaps I would have learned something important about age norms had I told her and had the opportunity to hear her reactions. On the other hand, perhaps she would have felt that the divide between us was too great and been more inhibited in my presence. As with all dilemmas, there are pros and cons to our decisions. (Edin and Kefalas, 2005, likewise mused on this issue in their book describing their research with low-income families.)

Professional Development Dilemma for Qualitative Researchers

I end with a caveat for young researchers—in my field and, I am told, in related social science fields, there are professional penalties that work against those who solely employ qualitative research methods. It is still the case that qualitative pieces appear infrequently in top-tier journals in psychology and child development. The problem may be exacerbated for scholars involved in translational research because, as pointed out by Wethington and Pillemer (2007), the tenure clock does not make allowances for the time it takes to establish and maintain collaborative relationships in the community. Furthermore, in some circles, applied research is viewed as less rigorous than work based on tightly controlled experimental procedures.

On the other hand, respect for qualitative approaches has been enhanced by National Science Foundation and National Institutes of Health endorsements in the form of grant support and workshops convened to articulate standards for rigor in qualitative research (e.g., Lamont & White, 2005). Moreover, increasingly, researchers are calling for mixed methods (McCall & Green, 2004; Yoshikawa, Weisner, Kalil, & Way, 2008). Strong studies integrating qualitative and quantitative work can capture the advantages of both approaches and support researchers' chances for professional advancement. As I learned from the experience of a former graduate research assistant who easily achieved tenure at a major university, a dossier comprising a set of papers based on qualitative methods complemented by another set based on quantitative methods is likewise a viable route. Even more telling of a change in attitude is the appearance this past year of position announcements specifically asking for expertise in qualitative research. These are encouraging signs.

SUMMARY

Qualitative research methods, especially when used in conjunction with quantitative methods, have the potential to enhance our understanding of the impacts of societal, family, and program conditions on individual and family current and long-term functioning. They also lend themselves well to written reports that are interesting and accessible to policymakers, practitioners, and the public. However, a number of dilemmas in the conduct and publication of qualitative research methods should be acknowledged. Those discussed in this chapter can be divided into three sets. The first set involves ethical dilemmas that occur when researchers feel torn between the desire to report on conditions as they would play out if they did not intervene and their beliefs that they have a moral obligation to help. The second set involves challenges in managing seemingly close yet imbalanced relationships. The third set involves professional advancement problems that can beset the researcher who focuses solely on qualitative methods. Current calls for mixed methods in translational research would seem to offer opportunities to resolve these concerns.

REFERENCES

Administration on Children, Youth and Families. (1994). *The statement of the advisory committee on services for families with infants and toddlers*. Washington, DC: U.S. Department of Health and Human Services.

Administration for Children and Families. (2002a). *Making a difference in the lives of infants and toddlers and their families: The impacts of Early Head Start: Vol. I. Final Technical Report*. Washington, DC: U.S. Department of Health and Human Services.

Administration for Children and Families. (2002b). *Making a difference in the lives of infants and toddlers and their families: The impacts of Early Head Start: Vol. II. Final Technical Report Appendixes*. Washington, DC: U.S. Department of Health and Human Services.

Administration for Children and Families. (2006). *Preliminary results of the Early Head Start prekindergarten followup*. Washington, DC: U.S. Department of Health and Human Services.

Bazeley, P., & Richards, L. (2000). *The NVivo qualitative project book*. Thousand Oaks, CA: Sage.

Brookes, S., Summers, J. A., Thornburg, K., Ispa, J. M., & Lane, V. (2006). Building successful home visitor–mother relationships: A qualitative look at contributing factors. *Early Childhood Research Quarterly, 21*, 25–45. doi:10.1016/j.ecresq.2006.01.005

Brookes, S. J., Thornburg, K. R., & Ispa, J. M. (2006). Home visitor roles and dilemmas. In J. M. Ispa, K. R. Thornburg, & M. A. Fine (Eds.), *Keepin' on: The everyday struggles of young families in poverty* (pp. 249–266). Baltimore, MD: Brookes.

Cicirelli, V. G. (1969). *The impact of Head Start: An evaluation of the effects of Head Start on children's cognitive and affective development*. Washington, DC: National Bureau of Standards, Institute for Applied Technology.

Collins, P. H. (1990). *Black feminist thought*. Boston, MA: Unwin Hyman.

Creswell, J. W. (1998). *Qualitative inquiry and research design: Choosing among five traditions*. Thousand Oaks, CA: Sage.

Deater-Deckard, K., & Dodge, K. A. (1997). Externalizing behavior problems and discipline revisited: Nonlinear effects and variation by culture, context, and gender. *Psychological Inquiry, 8,* 161–175. doi:10.1207/s15327965pli0803_1

Duneier, M. (1992). *Slim's table: Race, respectability, and masculinity.* Chicago, IL: University of Chicago Press.

Edin, K., & Kefalas, M. J. (2005). *Promises I can keep: Why poor women put motherhood before marriage.* Berkeley, CA: University of California Press.

Giles-Sims, J., Straus, M. A., & Sugarman, D. B. (1995). Child, maternal, and family characteristics associated with spanking. *Family Relations, 44,* 170–176. doi:10.2307/584804

Green, B. L., Mulvey, L., Fisher, H. A., & Rudacille, F. (1996). Integrating program and evaluation values: A family support approach to evaluation. *Evaluation Practice, 17,* 261–272. doi:10.1016/S0886-1633(96)90006-9

Hill, S. A., & Zimmerman, M. K. (1995). Valiant girls and vulnerable boys: The impact of gender and race on mothers' caregiving for chronically-ill children. *Journal of Marriage & the Family, 57,* 43–53. doi:10.2307/353815

Huston, A. C. (2005). Connecting the science of child development to public policy. *Society for Research in Child Development Social Policy Report, 19*(4), 1–18.

Ispa, J. M. (2002). Russian child care goals and values: From Perestroika to 2001. *Early Childhood Research Quarterly, 17,* 393–413. doi:10.1016/S0885-2006(02)00171-0

Ispa, J. M., Fine, M. A., Halgunseth, L. C., Harper, S., Robinson, J., Boyce, L., . . . Brady-Smith, C. (2004). Maternal intrusiveness, maternal warmth, and mother–toddler relationship outcomes: Variations across low-income ethnic and acculturation groups. *Child Development, 75,* 1613–1631. doi:10.1111/j.1467-8624.2004.00806.x

Ispa, J. M., & Halgunseth, L. C. (2004). Talking about corporal punishment: Nine low-income African American mothers' perspectives. *Early Childhood Research Quarterly, 19,* 463–484. doi:10.1016/j.ecresq.2004.07.002

Ispa, J. M., & Sharp, E. A. (2006). Andreya: An in-depth case study. In J. M. Ispa, K. R. Thornburg, & M. A. Fine (Eds.), *Keepin' on: The everyday struggles of young families in poverty* (pp. 35–107). Baltimore, MD: Brookes.

Ispa, J. M., Thornburg, K. R., & Fine, M. A. (2006). *Keepin' on: The everyday struggles of young families in poverty.* Baltimore, MD: Brookes.

Kvale, S. (1996). *An introduction to qualitative research interviewing.* Thousand Oaks, CA: Sage.

Lamont, M., & White, P. (2005). *Workshop on interdisciplinary standards for systematic qualitative research.* Report of a workshop supported by the National Science Foundation. Retrieved from http://www.nsf.gov/sbe/ses/soc/ISSQR_workshop_rpt.pdf

Love, J. M., Kisker, E. E., Ross, C., Raikes, H., Constantine, J., Boller, K., . . . Vogel C. (2005). The effectiveness of Early Head Start for 3-year-old children and their parents: Lessons for policy and programs. *Developmental Psychology, 41,* 885–901. doi:10.1037/0012-1649.41.6.885

Maccoby, E. E., Kahn, A. J., & Everett, B. A. (1983). The role of psychological research in the formation of policies affecting children. *American Psychologist, 38,* 80–84. doi:10.1037/0003-066X.38.1.80

McCall, R. B. (2009). Evidence-based programming in the context of policy and practice. *Society for Research in Child Development Social Policy Report, 23*(3), 1–19.

McCall, R. B., & Green, B. L. (2004). Beyond the methodological gold standards of behavioral research: Considerations for public policy. *Society for Research in Child Development Social Policy Report, 18*(2), 1–19.

Merrick, E. (1999). "Like chewing gravel": On the experience of analyzing qualitative research findings using a feminist epistemology. *Psychology of Women Quarterly, 23,* 47–57. doi:10.1111/j.1471-6402.1999.tb00340.x

Moffitt, R. (2000, January/February). Perspectives on the qualitative–quantitative divide. *Poverty Research News, 4,* 5–6.

Musick, J., & Stott, F. (2000). Paraprofessionals revisited and reconsidered. In J. P. Shonkoff & S. J. Meisels (Eds.), *Handbook of early childhood intervention* (2nd ed., pp. 439–453). New York, NY: Cambridge University Press.

Myerhoff, B. (1978). *Number our days.* New York, NY: Simon & Schuster.

National Association for the Education of Young Children & Society for Research in Child Development. (2008). Using research to improve outcomes for young children: A call for action: Final report of the Wingspread Conference, September 18–20, 2007. *Early Childhood Research Quarterly, 23,* 591–596. doi:10.1016/j.ecresq.2008.08.004

Patton, M. Q. (1990). *Qualitative research and evaluation methods* (2nd ed.). Newbury Park, CA: Sage.

Raikes, H. H., Pan, B., Luze, G., Tamis-LeMonda, C., Brooks-Gunn, J., Tarullo, L., . . . Rodriguez, E. (2006). Mother–child bookreading in low-income families: Predictors and outcomes during the first three years of life. *Child Development, 77,* 924–953. doi:10.1111/j.1467-8624.2006.00911.x

Richards, L., & Morse, J. M. (2007). *Read me first for a user's guide to qualitative methods* (2nd ed.). Thousand Oaks, CA: Sage Publications.

Rubin, H., & Rubin, I. (1995). *Qualitative interviewing: The art of hearing data.* Thousand Oaks, CA: Sage.

Sharp, E. A., & Ispa, J. M. (2009). Inner-city single black mothers' gender-related childrearing expectations and goals. *Sex Roles, 60,* 656–668. doi:10.1007/s11199-008-9567-3

Sharp, E. A., Ispa, J. M., Thornburg, K. R., & Lane, V. (2003). Relations among mother and home visitor personality, relationship quality, and amount of time spent in home visits. *Journal of Community Psychology, 31,* 591–606. doi:10.1002/jcop.10070

Shonkoff, J. P., & Phillips, D. A. (Eds.). (2000). *From neurons to neighborhoods: The science of early childhood development.* Washington, DC: National Academies Press.

Strauss, A., & Corbin, J. (1998). *Basics of qualitative research: Techniques and procedures for developing grounded theory* (2nd ed.). Thousand Oaks, CA: Sage.

Thompson, L. (1992). Feminist methodology for family studies. *Journal of Marriage and Family, 54,* 3–18. doi:10.2307/353271

Wethington, E., & Pillemer, K. A. (2007, Winter). Translating basic research into community practice: The Cornell Institute for Translational Research on Aging (CITRA). *Forum on Public Policy Online.* Retrieved from http://www.forumon publicpolicy.com

Wood, D., Kaplan, R., & McLoyd, V. C. (2007). Gender differences in the educational expectations of urban, low-income African American youth: The role of parents and the school. *Journal of Youth and Adolescence, 36,* 417–427. doi:10.1007/s10964-007-9186-2

Wuest, J. (1995). Feminist grounded theory: An exploration of the congruency and tensions between two traditions in knowledge discovery. *Qualitative Health Research, 5*(1), 125–138. doi:10.1177/104973239500500109

Yoshikawa, H., Weisner, T. S., Kalil, A., & Way, N. (2008). Mixing qualitative and quantitative methods in developmental science: Uses and methodological choices. *Developmental Psychology, 44,* 344–354. doi:10.1037/0012-1649.44.2.344

Zigler, E., & Muenchow, S. (1992). *Head Start: The inside story of America's most successful educational experiment.* New York, NY: Basic Books.

6

TRANSLATIONAL RESEARCH ON WORK AND FAMILY: DAILY STRESS PROCESSES IN HOTEL EMPLOYEES AND THEIR FAMILIES

DAVID M. ALMEIDA, KELLY D. DAVIS, JOHN W. O'NEILL, AND ANN C. CROUTER

Translational science calls on researchers to transform scientific discoveries into practical real-life applications. This chapter describes how we have been attempting to translate our research on work and family stressors to better understand and enhance the daily lives of hotel employees and their families. The Hotel Work and Well-Being Study involves the collaboration between an interdisciplinary team of investigators and hotel industry leaders, and hotel employees and their families. A major feature of this enterprise has been the application of the results from innovative methods of daily stress

This research was supported by the Alfred P. Sloan Foundation and conducted as part of the Work, Family and Health Network (http://www.WorkFamilyHealthNetwork.org), which is funded by a cooperative agreement through the National Institutes of Health and the Centers for Disease Control and Prevention: National Institute of Child Health and Human Development (NICHD; Grant # U01HD051217, U01HD051218, U01HD051256, U01HD051276), National Institute on Aging (Grant # U01AG027669), Office of Behavioral and Science Sciences Research, and National Institute for Occupational Safety and Health (Grant # U01OH008788). The contents of this publication are solely the responsibility of the authors and do not necessarily represent the official views of these institutes and offices. Special acknowledgment goes to extramural staff science collaborators Rosalind Berkowitz King and Lynne Casper for design of the original NICHD Workplace, Family, Health and Well-Being Network Initiative. We also appreciate the many insights of our hotel project collaborators, including Jan Cleveland, Laura Klein, Susan McHale, Amy Snead, and Courtney Whetzel.

research to the specific concerns of hotel employees and stakeholders with regard to work–family conflict.

The project has evolved through stages that exemplify important features of translational science. These stages include establishing close collaborations and dynamic feedback with important stakeholders, using the information obtained to design a study of daily stress and health specific to the hotel industry, disseminating findings to the industry stakeholders, and adapting knowledge gained in the process to evaluate a workplace program to alleviate the effects of work–family conflict on workers and their family members. This chapter uses examples of these activities to highlight multiple forms of translation.

DEVELOPING COLLABORATIVE RELATIONSHIPS WITH INDUSTRY STAKEHOLDERS

Our research aims to understand the predictors and consequences of work–family conflict. *Work–family conflict* is the extent to which fulfilling the responsibilities of both work and family roles is incompatible. This conflict could be rooted in time, strain, and/or behavior (Greenhaus & Beutell, 1985). Conflict could arise between the roles of worker and family member when one role is usurping time needed for the other role, such as long work hours reducing time spent at home with a spouse and children. Conflict can also arise when strain produced by one role makes performing another role difficult. For example, stressors at work can drain employees physically and mentally so that when they return home they withdraw or feel distant from family inter- actions. Finally, behaviors that are acceptable in one role may conflict with the norms and expectations for another role. For example, maternal behaviors, such as nurturing, may be valued less in the corporate work culture. Thus, being both a worker and a family member can create conflicts in life in several ways. This conflict between work and family, in turn, may have implications for health.

Several studies have investigated the link between experiences of work–family conflict and employee health. Work–family conflict has been associated with reports of poorer physical health (Dmitrieva, Baytalskaya, & Almeida, 2007; Frone, Russell, & Barnes, 1996; Grandey & Cropanzano, 1999), greater number of physical health symptoms (e.g., Adams & Jex, 1999; Netemeyer, Boles, & McMurrian, 1996), more chronic illnesses (Dmitrieva et al., 2007), heavier alcohol use (Frone et al., 1996), higher cholesterol (Thomas & Ganster, 1995), greater job burnout (Netemeyer et al., 1996), and greater work and family distress (Frone, Russell, & Cooper, 1992; Frone, Yardley, & Markel, 1997; Grandey & Cropanzano, 1999). Some studies have failed to establish the association between work–family conflict and health, such as Frone, Russell, and Cooper's (1997) 4-year longitudinal study of work–family conflict and employee health and hypertension. The majority of studies have, however, demonstrated a link between work–family conflict and employee health.

Employees' work–family conflict can influence the work–family experiences of other family members as well as their health. Research has demonstrated that one spouse's work–family conflict can be positively associated with the other spouse's work–family conflict (Cinamon, Weisel, & Tzuk, 2007; Hammer, Allen, & Grigsby, 1997; Westman & Etzion, 2005). This is a form of stress crossover, which is an interindividual process linking the stresses and strains of the worker to outcomes for another person, such as a spouse or child (Westman, 2001). Some studies have examined how employees' experiences of work–family conflict have implications for family members' health. For example, McLoyd, Toyokawa, and Kaplan (2008), looking at a sample of African American families, linked parents' work demands to increased work–family conflict, leading ultimately to increased externalizing behavior problems among children. More studies examining how work–family conflict experiences of one family member can influence the health and well-being of other members are needed. Furthermore, many of the studies examining work–family conflict have used heterogeneous community samples with little to no connection with specific industries. Within-industry research is vital in understanding how work experiences can influence employee health and family members' health.

In an effort to integrate a more focused and practical approach to work–family conflict, we received a program officer's grant from the Alfred P. Sloan Foundation to learn about work and family issues in the hotel industry (Cleveland, O'Neill, Crouter, & Drago, 2004). The goals of this effort were (a) to create an advisory council of industry leaders; (b) to gather pilot data that would provide insights about industry-specific work–family themes; and (c) to build a cohesive, multidisciplinary team for future collaborations.

Connecting With Stakeholders: Industry Leaders

Because we believed it important to have access to the views of opinion makers in the industry, our project team established the Hotels and Home Lives Advisory Council. Seven highly placed industry leaders graciously agreed to serve as a sounding board for our research planning. The council convened in January 2004 at the headquarters of the American Hotel & Lodging Association in Washington, DC. Members had a range of expertise; the group included a director of human resources of a large urban hotel, the president of the American Hotel & Lodging Association, the senior director of workplace strategies at Marriott, the CEO for Corporate Voices for Working Families, and CEOs and vice presidents of hospitality organizations. Council members provided frank advice, encouraging some research directions and questioning others. Council feedback greatly enhanced our understanding of the unique characteristics and needs of the hotel industry as they pertained to work–family conflict.

What We Learned

The American hotel industry is a large and growing segment of the U.S. economy, a sector in which many of the issues that characterize modern workplaces are particularly acute. Hotels operate on a 24-hour/7-day-a-week basis, including holidays. On the one hand, the industry's narrow profit margin leads to lean staffing patterns with many employees working long, often unpredictable hours. On the other hand, the 24/7 nature of the business may also provide opportunities for innovative employee schedule flexibility models that have the potential to improve worker and family health.

Since the terrorist attacks of September 11, 2001, and the subsequent precipitous drop in travel, hotel companies have faced difficult economic challenges and, as a result, have learned to do more with less. This challenge was exacerbated during the recent recession, which hit the hospitality industry hard. Lean staffing structures have placed heavy demands on hotel employees, which may, in turn, pose challenges for their physical and psychological health, work performance and productivity, and lives off the job (Mulvaney, O'Neill, Cleveland, & Crouter, 2007). One of the primary objectives of hotel companies is customer service, which means employees must react professionally and courteously to unexpected negative interactions with guests, interactions that often require significant emotion management (Grandey, Tam, & Brauburger, 2002). The hotel industry has high turnover due to several characteristics, including the frequent relocation of employees, in addition to the 24/7 operations. The median annual turnover rate for management positions is 21% and for nonmanagement positions is 50% (Smith Travel Research, 2003). Among the reasons employees quit their jobs in the hotel industry are work–family conflicts, that is, not having enough time to spend with their families due to the demands of the job (Stalcup & Pearson, 2001).

Connecting With Stakeholders: Hotel Managers and Spouses

We also conducted in-depth, open-ended interviews with approximately 30 hotel middle managers employed in full-service hotels in metro areas on the East Coast and with their spouses. Our racially and ethnically diverse sample of managers included men and women from different companies and in operations and nonoperations positions, including managers of food and beverage, rooms, marketing, accounting, engineering, and human resources. All couples had at least one child age 12 or under. Managers and spouses were interviewed separately, at home, in concurrent 2-hour sessions. These interviews were taped and subsequently transcribed.

What We Learned

Middle managers described a combination of positive and negative work conditions. On the one hand, they underscored the close relationships they had formed at work and the family-like climate and party atmosphere in many hotels, an atmosphere dependent in part on the attitudes, management style, and flexibility of the hotel general manager supervising them. (The general manager oversees the middle managers and hourly employees for all areas of a hotel.) Middle managers appreciated sharing some benefits, such as discounted vacation hotel rooms and free meals, with their families and exposing their children to a cosmopolitan lifestyle. The predominant negative themes pertained to time, especially long and often unpredictable hours at work and frequent weekends and holidays away from home. If issues arose at the hotel that needed their attention, the managers had to stay longer or come into the hotel. Pagers and cell phones created permeable work–family boundaries, making it difficult ever to feel completely away from work. Some middle managers also suggested that the long work hours, coupled with the hotel industry's party atmosphere, contributed to substance abuse, infidelity, and divorce. Another contributor to work strain was the need to respond professionally to angry guests. Following days that involved emotionally arousing encounters, middle managers described either withdrawing temporarily from family interaction or letting off steam. A less frequently mentioned theme was the challenges that work-imposed geographic moves created for families. Interestingly, couples described the work–family interface more positively when the spouse had firsthand employment experience in the industry.

Although we were not funded to study hourly employees in this research, many middle managers provided examples of ways in which their work lives were affected adversely by the ongoing work and family challenges experienced by the hourly employees (e.g., housekeeping, food and beverage, and front desk staff) they supervised. Hourly employee tardiness and absenteeism, for example, created ripple effects throughout the hotel work context as others had to fill in or adjust accordingly. This situation underscores the importance of learning more not only about the work and family lives of hotel managers but also about the work and nonwork experiences of hourly employees, as well as how the work experiences of these two important groups intersect.

INCORPORATING EMPLOYEES' NEEDS AND
CONCERNS INTO A STUDY

Our discussions with industry leaders as well as with hotel middle managers and their spouses indicated that some common stressors may be linked to the health of managers and possibly of their family members, including long and unpredictable work hours; schedules that do not dovetail well with family schedules, routines, and rituals (e.g., weekend, holiday work); permeable family boundaries (e.g., pagers, cell phones); unexpected problems that require immediate attention (e.g., overbooked rooms, absent employees); and stressful interactions with guests and coworkers that must be handled professionally (Cleveland et al., 2004).

Building on this information, we were funded by the Eunice Kennedy Shriver National Institute of Child Health and Human Development (NICHD) to be a part of the Work, Family & Health Network to carry out a larger and more systematic study of the effects of daily stress on hotel employees and their family members. This project collects information using daily diaries as a tool for understanding the work–family interface in its dynamic complexity. In particular, this project highlights our group's interest in understanding the day-to-day processes through which daily stressors on the job come to shape the daily health and well-being of individual hotel employees and their spouses or partners. A unique feature of the research is the combination of daily self-reports of work and family experiences and physiological indicators of heath, assessed via salivary cortisol sampling. We argue that the daily diary method is an essential tool for translational research focused on work and family because it can illuminate, on a day-to-day basis, how the dual responsibilities of work and family life can lead to daily indicators of work–family conflict and to perceived and physiological health.

Conceptual Background

We designed the project to be a telephone diary study of daily stressors and health among hotel hourly workers and their children and middle managers and their spouses. The primary goal was to examine patterns of exposure to day-to-day work and family stressors as well as individuals' physical and emotional reactivity to these stressors. *Daily stressors* are defined as relatively minor events arising out of day-to-day living, such as the everyday concerns of work, caring for others, and commuting between work and home. They can also refer to small, unexpected events that disrupt daily life: "little" life events, such as arguments with children, unexpected work deadlines, or a malfunctioning computer (Almeida, 2005). Several studies have found that the frequency and type of daily stressors provide a better explanation for short-term psychological and somatic health outcomes than do major life events in the recent past or chronic, role-related stressors (Bolger, DeLongis, Kessler, & Schilling, 1989; Eckenrode, 1984; Lazarus, 1984).

Advantages of Daily Diary Methods

The understanding of daily stressors has benefited from the development of diary methods that involve repeated measurements on individuals during their daily lives (Almeida, 2005). On each occasion of measurement, individuals report the stressors they experienced on that day as well as the behaviors, physical symptoms, and emotional states they experienced during that same time frame. Paper and pencil diaries have been criticized for potential lack of compliance on the part of some participants in completing diaries at scheduled times (Stone, Shiffman, Schwartz, Broderick, & Hufford, 2002). Recent diary methods, such as telephone interviews, PDAs, and Internet web pages, however, provide more control over compliance and allow for more in-depth information through skip patterns and open-ended probes. Diary methods have a number of other virtues (Bolger, Davis, & Rafaeli, 2003). Obtaining information about individuals' actual daily stressors over short-term intervals circumvents concerns about ecological validity that constrain findings from laboratory research. Furthermore, diary methods alleviate memory distortions, which can occur in more traditional questionnaire and interview methods, that require respondents to recall experiences over longer time frames.

Perhaps the most valuable feature of diary methods is the ability to assess within-person processes. This paradigm represents a shift from identifying universal, between-person patterns of association between stressors and health to charting the day-to-day fluctuations in stress and health within individuals as well as identifying their predictors, correlates, and sequelae (Reis & Gable, 2000). Stress is a process that occurs within the individual, and research designs need to reflect this. The unique advantages of a diary approach can lead to significant contributions to the literature on the health effects of work–family conflict (Perry-Jenkins, Repetti, & Crouter, 2000). For example, instead of asking whether individuals with high levels of work–family conflict experience more physical health problems than individuals with less stressful jobs, a researcher can ask whether a worker experiences more health problems on days when he or she has too many deadlines (or is reprimanded) than on days when work has been stress free. Importantly, this within-person approach allows the researcher to rule out stable personality and environmental factors as third-variable explanations for the relation between stressors and health. In addition, the intensive longitudinal aspect of this design permits a temporal examination of how stressors are associated with changes in health from one day to the next. By establishing within-person through-time associations between daily stressors and health, researchers can more precisely establish the short-term effects of specific daily experiences (Bolger et al., 2003; Larson & Almeida, 1999). As we will underscore in our concluding remarks about this project, we think this feature has enormous potential for understanding how workplace interventions work on a daily basis.

Advantages of Salivary Assessments of Health

We have extended our analysis of daily physical health by collecting multiple daily samples of saliva that are assayed for diurnal cortisol. Diurnal cortisol is a biological marker of activity of the hypothalamic-pituitary-adrenal (HPA) axis. The HPA axis plays a vital role in linking stressor exposure to physical health (McEwen, 1998), as cortisol can affect many biological systems essential to normal functioning. Many studies have documented elevated cortisol levels in response to laboratory-controlled acute psychological stressors (Dickerson & Kemeny, 2004). Much less is known about the links between naturally occurring stressors and cortisol (cf. Almeida, McGonagle, & King, 2009; Dettenborn et al., 2005; Polk, Cohen, Doyle, Skoner, & Kirschbaum, 2005). Our research examines diurnal patterns in salivary cortisol, which typically peak shortly after waking in the morning and gradually decline throughout the day. Diurnal cortisol permits a view into individual chronobiology (Keenan, Licinio, & Veldhuis, 2001). If the cortisol rhythm becomes disrupted, other biological rhythms may also become dysregulated, including lymphocyte production, basal body temperature, and sleep (Cugini, Romit, di Palma, & Giacovazzo, 1990). Examining patterns of cortisol throughout the day provides a window into the extent to which the HPA axis is responding to the external environment. Failure to activate the HPA axis in the morning or deactivate it in the evening may indicate a difficulty in disengaging from external demands, leading to inhibition of restoration and recovery processes (Sapolsky, Krey, & McEwen, 1986). Studying cortisol in the field allows us to examine how daily life experiences—such as those in the workplace—influence daily physiology and are associated with indicators of health and well-being.

We also take the innovative step of examining how parents' daily experiences are linked to their children's daily stress physiology and health. The effects of work–family conflict are not limited to the individual. Family members and close others may also bear the brunt of such stressors. Larson and Almeida (1999) proposed a research paradigm to assess emotional transmission in families. Within this paradigm the family is viewed as a nexus of daily interchanges among household members and between these members and the world outside the family. Through regular patterns of interactions with each other and outside systems, family members are affected by and affect each other. The project focused primarily on how the work setting affects not only the employee's health but also the child's or spouse's health (i.e., crossover) and other indicators of family functioning. For example, a worker experiencing a great deal of interpersonal tension at work may experience psychological distress that is brought home in the evening and regularly affects her spouse and children. Through such chain reactions, stressors enter the family through a particular family member and are transmitted to other family members in a predictable sequence.

In summary, using information gained from hotel employees and industry stakeholders and funds from the Sloan Foundation and NICHD, we designed a diary study that addresses their concerns and seeks to uncover how work–family conflict is linked to health and family relationships on a day-to-day basis. Understanding how these experiences are linked at a more fine-grained level can allow for greater specification of workplace programs and interventions.

Summary of Study Methodology and Key Findings

Our research has focused on the experiences of hotel employees, including the daily work experiences of individuals in different positions in the industry (middle managers, hourly workers). After hotel general managers were interviewed on-site, 77% gave us permission to contact their middle managers, of whom 86% ($N = 588$) agreed to be in the study and complete a telephone interview. We asked to do a telephone interview with the manager's spouse or partner where applicable, and 197 agreed. To recruit hourly employees and one of their children (ages 10–18), we requested permission from human resources managers at hotels across the United States to have research assistants set up tables (usually in the staff cafeteria at the hotel) to share information about the Hotel Work and Well-Being Study. As a result, 157 hourly employees expressed an interest in participating. Of the 105 eligible participants (hourly employee, proficient in English, had a child in the age range), 75 (71%) completed a baseline telephone survey. (Middle managers, their spouses, and hourly employees completed the baseline survey; children did not.)

Hotel employees who completed the baseline survey were asked whether they would be willing to participate with their respective family member in a daily diary study. We examined work–family processes by measuring daily experiences of 98 managers and 42 of their partners and 66 hourly hotel workers and their offspring (ages 10–18). Middle managers (female = 48%, White = 68%) who participated in the daily diary were, on average, 38 years old, had some college education, and had been in the hospitality industry for 13 years. They had a median income of $58,240 (range = $24,000–$120,000), and 58% were parents. Managers' spouses or partners were 37 years old and had some college education, on average. Eighty-one percent were employed, and 30% had worked or were currently working at a hotel. Hourly employees who completed the daily diary were mostly African American (65%) mothers (80%) who were 40 years old with nearly 10 years of experience in the industry, on average. Hourly participants included housekeeping, food and beverage, and front desk staff. Their median income was $26,194 (range = $1,525–$45,000). The children (45% female) who participated in the diary were almost 14 years old ($M = 13.69$, $SD = 2.31$), on average.

Hotel employees and their family members were telephoned on 8 consecutive days and asked to report on their daily experiences, including time use, stressful experiences, family processes, and daily psychological and physical well-being. On 4 of those days they also were asked to provide saliva samples at four points during the day (upon waking, 30 minutes after waking, before lunch, and at bedtime). These samples were assayed for cortisol. Data from this research provide compelling evidence of the health effects of work–family conflict by establishing links between daily stressors and daily well-being in workers and their families.

What We Learned: Prevalence of Daily Workplace Stressors and Daily Health

Daily Stress and Health Measures

Across the 8 interview days, compared with hourly employees, middle managers reported more arguments at work (13% vs. 7% of the days), interpersonal tensions (23% vs. 11%), stressors involving employees and coworkers (14% vs. 4%), hotel guest stressors (9% vs. 3%), and work overloads (e.g., equipment breakdowns; 20% vs. 8%; O'Neill & Davis, 2011). Middle managers reported, on average across the 8 days, two health symptoms (e.g., headache, stomachache) a day (range = 0–18) and low negative affect ($M = 0.26$, $SD = 0.24$), that is, on average they were not upset, nervous, or afraid. Hourly employees mirrored this pattern.

Work can "get under the skin" by affecting emotional and physiological processes (Taylor, Repetti, & Seeman, 1997). For example, preliminary analyses revealed that, on days when middle managers had interpersonal work stressors, they also reported higher negative affect ($\gamma = 0.15$, $p < .001$) and more physical health problems ($\gamma = 0.52$, $p < .01$). Hourly employees followed the same pattern, reporting greater negative affect ($\gamma = 0.10$, $p < .01$) and more health symptoms ($\gamma = 0.81$, $p < .001$) on interpersonal work stressor days compared with nonstressor days.

Daily work experiences were also linked to the daily rhythm of cortisol across the 4 days of assessment according to the results of a three-level (cortisol collections within day, days within persons) model that focused on

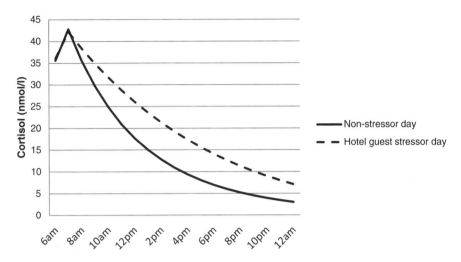

Figure 6.1. Diurnal rhythm of hotel managers' cortisol on days with and without hotel guest stressors.

two components of the diurnal cortisol pattern: the morning rise and daily decline throughout the day. Interpersonal work stressors were associated with the change in the rate of the decline (i.e., quadratic effect). Figure 6.1 shows the within-person effects. These analyses are based on up to 16 observations per individual, collected on work- and nonworkdays, allowing us to achieve reliable estimates of change across the day. Our findings show that, on days when managers reported having interpersonal stressors, the rate of their decline was less steep than usual, indicating that their stress hormones remained elevated throughout the day.

Work-to-Family Spillover and Crossover

Our design also allows us to examine stress processes that occur within individuals and family. We can examine *work–family spillover*, an intra-individual process in which experiences at work transfer (or spill over) to nonwork areas (namely, the family) and vice versa (Staines, 1980). We can also examine *crossover*, an interindividual process in which the experiences and strain of one person are connected to those of another (Westman, 2001). By studying these processes on a daily basis, we illuminate how work stressors influence employee and child health.

Preliminary analyses with our hotel sample demonstrate the power of a diary design to capture both of these processes. Compared with typical workdays, for example, male middle managers reported spending less time with their children on days when the parents had interpersonal work stressors

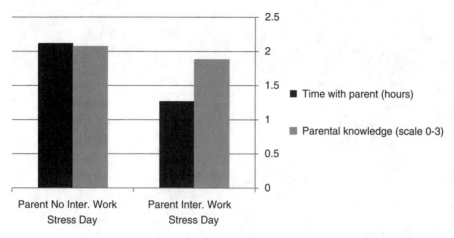

Figure 6.2. Children's report of parents' time with them and knowledge on days with and without interpersonal work stressors. Both results are significant at *p* < .05.

($\gamma = -1.85, p < .01$). In addition, managers (both male and female) spent less time with their children on days they spent more time at work ($\gamma = -0.26, p < .001$). In these analyses, the significant differences were not between managers but reflect differences within managers from one day to the next.

Daily work stressors were linked to children's reports of parenting and family life as well. Similar results emerged when using child reports of time with their hourly hotel parents. Figure 6.2 shows that children reported spending nearly 1 hour less with their parents on days when their parents had an interpersonal work stressor and 20 minutes less when parents had to work longer than normal. Also shown in Figure 6.2 is that children reported that their working parents knew less about what the children did on days when they had interpersonal stressors at work. On days when parents stayed longer at work, children reported that their parents knew less about their whereabouts and experiences that day. Consistent with the idea that children can be affected by "secondhand emotion" (Larson & Almeida, 1999), on days when mothers had interpersonal work stressors, boys had lower positive affect than on days when mothers did not have these stressors (Davis, 2008).

In summary, this work provides detailed assessment of how work stressors in the hotel industry affect not only workers but also their interactions with children. Through our discussions and qualitative interviews we were able to learn a great deal about potential sources of stress in hotels and its potential impact on hotel workers. This information was vital in our design of a study that assessed how work and family conflict unfold on a daily basis as well as in understanding how such stressors affect the health and well-being of workers and family members. The next step in our research program was to translate these findings for use in the hotel industry.

DISSEMINATING FINDINGS AND RECOMMENDATIONS TO STAKEHOLDERS

A major aim of this project was to disseminate our findings and recommendations to hotel industry leaders and to the industry as whole. We take the goal of putting the research findings into industry hands very seriously. Toward that goal, we have conducted presentations at hotel industry conferences and shows; provided newsletters to our advisory council, general managers, and executives; and created a glossy report to send to all parties who were involved or who expressed an interest in the project.

Hotel Industry Shows

We presented information from our study at four hotel shows, including two presentations at Army Lodging meetings and a presentation at the Pennsylvania Tourism and Lodging Association Annual Conference. Our team was the first to present empirical work–family scholarship at a hotel show, including the most prestigious of its kind—the International Hotel, Motel, and Restaurant Show held in New York City in November, 2007. The presentations provided an overview of the project, preliminary findings, and action ideas. The focus was on how to recruit and retain talent—two major concerns in the hotel industryby understanding how work in the hospitality industry can enhance or reduce the quality of life on and off the job. Findings included how workplace characteristics, such as the leadership style of general managers and how supportive the climate is for managing work and family responsibilities, were linked to managers' perceptions of negative work–family spillover and turnover intentions. Examples of action ideas presented to the hotel industry audience were (a) to invest in leadership development, (b) to use flexibility as compensation for managers who have little control over their work hours, and (c) to enculturate spouses or partners so that they understand the industry and the effects it can have on managers. All the shows were attended by hundreds of hotel industry executives and managers, who were actively engaged in discussions surrounding the issues presented. The hotel shows allowed us to bring information directly to the industry.

Newsletters

In addition to presenting information at the hotel shows, we disseminated information about the study to members of the hotel industry via newsletters. When we had sufficient participation at the hotel level, we provided general managers with a customized report that compared the means on certain key work–family indicators for their hotel versus the sample as a whole. The individualized reports showed how their hotel compared with the rest of the sample on various indices, such as job satisfaction, burnout, work–family culture, turnover, job demands, and work–family spillover. We also sent three one-page newsletters to the advisory council, hotel executives, general managers, and middle managers who participated, periodically updating them regarding the progress of the study (e.g., number of completed interviews, next steps). These newsletters were sent to more than 600 people in the hotel industry.

Report to Stakeholders

We created a glossy, bound report that highlights the findings from the hotel study to date and provides a list of recommendations for the hotel industry (http://www.hhdev.psu.edu/HotelProject/). The report is for the advisory council members as well as hotel executives, general managers, middle managers, spouses or partners, and hourly employees who participated in the study. The following recommendations are based on the results of our project. They are intended to help hotel organizations develop workplace policies and practices that promote employee health, retention, and productivity.

Provide Flexibility as Compensation to Employees

Although traditional pay and benefits are important components of employee compensation packages, we discovered that hotel workers are increasingly citing work–family flexibility as important. For example, one hourly employee wanted schedule flexibility to go to a much-needed dentist appointment that had been postponed two times because of her work schedule. Furthermore, our research suggests that general managers who support work–family balance have employees who are more committed to their work and less likely to leave their current position.

Reduce Stress in the Workplace

Our research shows that hotel workers' well-being is better on stress-free days than on stressful days. Making hotel workers aware of the negative implications of work stress, as well as promoting positive coping strategies (e.g., conflict management), may improve employee well-being. Furthermore, when employee health is improved, job performance is likely improved as well.

Support Work–Family Balance for General Managers

Stress is contagious. We found that general managers with children experienced significantly more work-to-family stress than general managers without children. Furthermore, we found that the general manager's work and family stress can be felt throughout the entire hotel (O'Neill et al., 2009). Specifically, middle managers were less likely to think about leaving their jobs when their general manager experienced less negative work-to-family spillover. When general managers were more supportive of middle manager needs to balance work and family responsibilities, middle managers reported that they were more committed to their organization and less likely to consider leaving their organization for another job. Providing more support to general managers to help balance work and family responsibilities not only can reduce general manager levels of negative work-to-family spillover but also may help to create a culture in which all employees are supported in balancing work and family responsibilities.

Ensure That General Managers Send the Right Message to Employees

We found that work culture was linked to employee well-being, job performance, and intentions to leave the company. Leaders play a significant role in creating the work culture. Through the messages they send and by rewarding and encouraging certain behaviors, leaders can influence employees' perceptions of organizational culture. For example, general managers who take time to attend their children's events could foster a family-friendly atmosphere by setting an example for other managers to take time for family and by encouraging this behavior in others. It is important for general managers and other organizational leaders to send clear messages that let employees know the organization is supportive of employees' responsibilities both within and outside of the workplace and is committed to helping employees at all levels within the organization achieve better work–family balance.

APPLYING LESSONS LEARNED TO INTERVENTION EVALUATION

We have learned a great deal about doing industry-specific research, particularly studying a customer-driven, 24/7 industry. The lessons gleaned from the Hotel Work and Well-Being Study are now part of the foundation for a new collaborative study involving the NICHD Work, Family & Health Network. This project involves an investigation of the effects of an employer-initiated workplace program on employees, families, and children. The workplace program focuses on increasing employee flexibility and control over how and when their work is done and increasing support from supervisors and coworkers for employees' work–family issues. Companies in two industries are implementing the program, the IT/telecommunications industry and the extended care/nursing home industry. Although we will not be studying the hotel industry in this collaborative project, we are parlaying our experiences with that industry in many ways. Using the same daily diary method described above, we are conducting daily diary interviews with a subsample of employees and their children ages 9 to 17 before and 12 months after the program. The purpose of this aspect of the study is to test whether the effects of the program spill over to employees' global and daily family processes (e.g., marital satisfaction, parental involvement) and health (physical symptoms, biological indicators of daily stress) and cross over to improve global and daily health in spouses and children. This study will also incorporate the saliva collection method described above. The methodological innovations of our daily stress approach will contribute to the network's ability to better inform and assess workplace programs.

CONCLUSION

The overarching goal of translational science is to transform scientific discoveries into practical applications. In medicine, such discoveries typically begin at "the bench" and then progress to the clinical level, or the patient's "bedside." In the social sciences, basic research often starts with broad surveys with fairly heterogeneous samples then proceeds to real-life application in specific settings. The transformation of "survey to setting" has involved multiple layers of translation in our research program. The purpose of this chapter was to describe a daily stress approach for translational research on work and family. Using examples from the Hotel Work and Well-Being Study we described how we attempted to translate our research on work–family conflict to understand and enhance the daily lives of hotel employees and their families.

The project started with translation of information *between* our research team and invested stakeholders. This exchange was reciprocal and dynamic. Our advisory council and qualitative interviews provided vital information on the nature and concerns of the hotel industry revolving around work–family issues. We then translated this information to the design and implementation of a systematic study of daily stress among hotel employees and family members. Our findings were then translated back to our stakeholders with suggestions and recommendations to enhance work and family life in the hotel industry.

We believe that research translation should move beyond making recommendations. Scientific knowledge should also be translated into the development of theoretically based but practical interventions that are likely to succeed in addressing health issues. We hope that the examples from our work on the health effects of work–family conflict provide useful information for other basic social scientists and motivate them to consider ways to translate their programs of research.

REFERENCES

Adams, G. A., & Jex, S. M. (1999). Relationships between time management, control, work–family conflict, and strain. *Journal of Occupational Health Psychology, 4*, 72–77. doi:10.1037/1076-8998.4.1.72

Almeida, D. M. (2005). Resilience and vulnerability to daily stressors assessed via diary methods. *Current Directions in Psychological Science, 14*, 64–68. doi:10.1111/j.0963-7214.2005.00336.x

Almeida, D. M., McGonagle, K., & King, H. (2009). Assessing daily stress processes in social surveys by combining stressor exposure and salivary cortisol. *Biodemography and Social Biology, 55*, 219–237. doi:10.1080/19485560903382338

Bolger, N., Davis, A., & Rafaeli, E. (2003). Diary methods: Capturing life as it is lived. *Annual Review of Psychology, 54*, 579–616. doi:10.1146/annurev.psych.54.101601.145030

Bolger, N., DeLongis, A., Kessler, R. C., & Schilling, E. A. (1989). Effects of daily stress on negative mood. *Journal of Personality and Social Psychology, 57*, 808–818. doi:10.1037/0022-3514.57.5.808

Cinamon, R. G., Weisel, A., & Tzuk, K. (2007). Work–family conflict within the family. *Journal of Career Development, 34*, 79–100.

Cleveland, J., O'Neill, J., Crouter, A. C., & Drago, R. (2004). Hotels and home lives. *Final report to the Alfred P. Sloan Foundation.*

Cugini, P., Romit, A., di Palma, L., & Giacovazzo, M. (1990). Common migraine as a weekly and seasonal headache. *Chronobiology International, 7*, 467–469. doi:10.3109/07420529009059158

Davis, K. D. (2008). *Daily positive and negative work–family spillover and crossover between mothers and children.* Unpublished doctoral dissertation, The Pennsylvania State University University Park Campus.

Dettenborn, L., James, G. D., van Berge-Landry, H., Valdimarsdottir, H. B., Montgomery, G. H., & Bovjerg, D. H. (2005). Heightened cortisol responses to daily stress in working women at familial risk for breast cancer. *Biological Psychology, 69*, 167–179. doi:10.1016/j.biopsycho.2004.07.004

Dickerson, S. S., & Kemeny, M. E. (2004). Acute stressors and cortisol responses: A theoretical integration and synthesis of laboratory research. *Psychological Bulletin, 130*, 355–391. doi:10.1037/0033-2909.130.3.355

Dmitrieva, N., Baytalskaya, N., & Almeida, D. M. (2007, November). Longitudinal changes in work–family conflict predict changes in health. Poster presented at the 60th Annual Scientific Meeting of the Gerontological Society of America, San Francisco, CA.

Eckenrode, J. (1984). Impact of chronic and acute stressors on daily reports of mood. *Journal of Personality and Social Psychology, 46*, 907–918. doi:10.1037/0022-3514.46.4.907

Frone, M. R., Russell, M., & Barnes, G. M. (1996). Work–family conflict, gender, and health-related outcomes: A study of employed parents in two community samples. *Journal of Occupational Health Psychology, 1*, 57–69. doi:10.1037/1076-8998.1.1.57

Frone, M. R., Russell, M., & Cooper, M. L. (1992). Antecedents and outcomes of work–family conflict: Testing a model of the work–family interface. *Journal of Applied Psychology, 77*, 65–78. doi:10.1037/0021-9010.77.1.65

Frone, M. R., Russell, M., & Cooper, M. L. (1997). Relation of work–family conflict to health outcomes: A four-year longitudinal study of employed parents. *Journal of Occupational and Organizational Psychology, 70*, 325–335. doi:10.1111/j.2044-8325.1997.tb00652.x

Frone, M. R., Yardley, J. K., & Markel, K. S. (1997). Developing an integrative model of the work–family interface. *Journal of Vocational Behavior, 50*, 145–167. doi:10.1006/jvbe.1996.1577

Grandey, A. A., & Cropranzano, R. (1999). The conservation of resource model applied to work–family conflict and strain. *Journal of Vocational Behavior, 54*, 350–370. doi:10.1006/jvbe.1998.1666

Grandey, A. A., Tam, A. P., & Brauburger, A. L. (2002). Affective states and traits in the workplace: Diary and survey data from young workers. *Motivation and Emotion, 26*, 31–55. doi:10.1023/A:1015142124306

Greenhaus, J. H., & Beutell, N. J. (1985). Sources of conflict between work and family roles. *Academy of Management Review, 10*, 78–88.

Hammer, L. B., Allen, E., & Grigsby, T. D. (1997). Work–family conflict in dual-earner couples: Within-individual and crossover effects of work and family. *Journal of Vocational Behavior, 50*, 185–203. doi:10.1006/jvbe.1996.1557

Keenan, D. M., Licinio, J., & Veldhuis, J. D. (2001). A feedback-controlled ensemble model of the stress-responsive hypothalamo-pituitary-adrenal axis. *Proceedings of the National Academy of Sciences of the United States of America, 98*, 4028–4033. doi:10.1073/pnas.051624198

Larson, R., & Almeida, D. M. (1999). Emotional transmission in the daily lives of families: A new paradigm for studying family process. *Journal of Marriage & the Family, 61*, 5–20. doi:10.2307/353879

Lazarus, R. S. (1984). Puzzles in the study of daily hassles. *Journal of Behavioral Medicine, 7*, 375–389. doi:10.1007/BF00845271

McEwen, B. S. (1998). Protective and damaging effects of stress mediators. *The New England Journal of Medicine, 338*, 171–179. doi:10.1056/NEJM199801153380307

McLoyd, V. C., Toyokawa, T., & Kaplan, R. (2008). Work demands, work–family conflict, and child adjustment in African American families: The mediating role of family routines. *Journal of Family Issues, 29,* 1247–1267. doi:10.1177/0192513X08320189

Mulvaney, R. H., O'Neill, J. W., Cleveland, J. N., & Crouter, A. C. (2007). A model of work and family dynamics hotel managers. *Annals of Tourism Research, 34,* 66–87.

Netemeyer, R. G., Boles, J. S., & McMurrian, R. (1996). Development and validation of work–family conflict and family–work conflict scales. *Journal of Applied Psychology, 81,* 400–410. doi:10.1037/0021-9010.81.4.400

O'Neill, J. W., & Davis, K. D. (2011). Work stress and well-being in the hotel industry. *International Journal of Hospitality Management, 30,* 385–390. doi:10.1016/j.ijhm.2010.07.007

O'Neill, J. W., Harrison, M. M., Cleveland, J. N., Almeida, D. M., Stawski, R. S., & Crouter, A. C. (2009). Work–family climate, organizational commitment, and turnover: Multilevel contagion effects of leaders. *Journal of Vocational Behavior, 74,* 18–29. doi:10.1016/j.jvb.2008.10.004

Perry-Jenkins, M., Repetti, R. L., & Crouter, A. C. (2000). Work and family in the 1990s. *Journal of Marriage & the Family, 62,* 981–998. doi:10.1111/j.1741-3737.2000.00981.x

Polk, D. E., Cohen, S., Doyle, W. J., Skoner, D. P., & Kirschbaum, C. (2005). State of trait and affect as predictors of salivary cortisol in healthy adults. *Psychoneuroendocrinology, 30,* 261–272. doi:10.1016/j.psyneuen.2004.08.004

Reis, H. T., & Gable, S. L. (2000). Event-sampling and other methods for studying everyday experience. In C. M. Judd & H. T. Reis (Eds.), *Handbook of research methods in social and personality psychology* (pp. 190–222). New York, NY: Cambridge University Press.

Sapolsky, R. M., Krey, L. C., & McEwen, B. S. (1986). The neuroendocrinology of stress and aging: The glucocorticoid cascade hypothesis. *Endocrine Reviews, 7,* 284–301. doi:10.1210/edrv-7-3-284

Smith Travel Research. (2003, March). *Announces Full Year 2002 U.S. Lodging Industry Results.* Retrieved from http://ehotelier.com/hospoitality-news/item.php?id=A871_0_11_0_M.

Staines, G. L. (1980). Spillover versus compensation: A review of the literature on the relationship between work and nonwork. *Human Relations, 33,* 111–129. doi:10.1177/001872678003300203

Stalcup, L. D., & Pearson, T. A. (2001). A model of the causes of management turnover in hotels. *Journal of Hospitality & Tourism Research, 25*(1), 17–30. doi:10.1177/109634800102500103

Stone, A. A., Shiffman, S., Schwartz, J. E., Broderick, J. E., & Hufford, M. R. (2002). Patient non-compliance with paper diaries. *British Medical Journal, 324,* 1193–1194. doi:10.1136/bmj.324.7347.1193

Taylor, S. E., Repetti, R. L., & Seeman, T. (1997). Health psychology: What is an unhealthy environment and how does it get under the skin? *Annual Review of Psychology, 48,* 411–447. doi:10.1146/annurev.psych.48.1.411

Thomas, L. T., & Ganster, D. C. (1995). Impact of family-supportive work variables on work–family conflict and strain: A control perspective. *Journal of Applied Psychology, 80*, 6–15. doi:10.1037/0021-9010.80.1.6

Westman, M. (2001). Stress and strain crossover. *Human Relations, 54*, 717–752. doi:10.1177/0018726701546002

Westman, M., & Etzion, D. (2005). The crossover of work–family conflict from one spouse to the other. *Journal of Applied Social Psychology, 35*, 1936–1957. doi:10.1111/j.1559-1816.2005.tb02203.x

7

THE SCIENCE OF LAW AND MEMORY

ERIC ZEMBER, CHARLES J. BRAINERD,
VALERIE F. REYNA, AND KIMBERLY A. KOPKO

This chapter focuses on the science of false memory and how it can be translated and applied to the law. We describe a major success story in the translation of basic psychological research to practice: the increasing influence of cognitive psychological findings about human memory and reasoning on the practice of law and the courts. Cognitive, social, and other research psychologists have influenced practices of police interrogation, preparation of witnesses for trial, evaluation of the validity of eyewitness testimony, and practices ensuring the credibility of child witnesses. We review new research findings on memory, suggestibility, decision making, evaluation of risks, and neuroscience that we believe constitute the next frontier in the translation of psychology to law and legal practice.

PSYCHOLOGY, MEMORY, AND THE LAW

Multiple events in the late 1980s and early 1990s brought to light some of the problems that can be caused by false memories. There was a recovered memory crisis in psychotherapy, wherein many individuals claimed to have exhumed repressed memories of being sexually abused and traumatized years before (often during childhood). In several high-profile cases, patients concluded that their memories were false and sued their therapist for having implanted them (Brainerd & Reyna, 2005). Research showed that certain features of psychotherapy compromise memory accuracy of traumatic experiences, and the courts, families, patients, and psychotherapists alike could not tell when reemerging memories were true and when they were false. In the same era, evidence came to light that many criminal investigations produce confessions, eyewitness identifications, and accusations that are all based on false memories (Brainerd & Reyna, 2005). When that evidence was combined with commonsense assumptions that the law makes about memory, the conclusion was that false memories can result in innocent people being prosecuted and the guilty going free and potentially reoffending (Reyna, Mills, Estrada, & Brainerd, 2007). These events made it necessary to develop a science of false memory to protect families, patients, and children.

The first two sections of this chapter provide background on the need for a translational science of false memory; the third delves into theoretical explanations of false memory that may be applied to the task of translation. We discuss how the science of false memory explains why and how false memories occur. To study false memory, researchers need to know which memories are false and which individuals are particularly vulnerable to them. The third section provides an overview of fuzzy trace theory's explanation of false memory (Brainerd, Reyna, & Ceci, 2008). We also discuss developmental reversals in false memory, which go against core assumptions that the law makes about memory. We note that some false memories increase as children develop, and in some cases, children's memories are actually more reliable than those of adults. In addition, we consider some key forgetting phenomena that elevate false memories.

The last section deals with translation to the law. The law's need for translational research is described in detail. Legal evidence is not like that depicted in the American police procedural *CSI* (*Crime Scene Investigation*) television series; physical evidence/forensic science is gathered in fewer than 10% of criminal cases in the United States (Horvath & Meesig, 1996, 1998). Legal evidence most often comes down to what people (witnesses, victims) can remember (during crime scene investigations, interviews, interrogations, eyewitness IDs, police reports, depositions, trial testimony), plus what people do with what they remember (judgment and decision making). If evidence in criminal investigations is mostly memory, then there is a critical need to understand why and how false memories infect evidence. Different areas of translational research in the law are discussed: The science of human memory is extensively examined, and brief consideration is given to the science of judgment and decision making. We highlight examples from the law where memory is fundamental to the evidence. We examine the accuracy and confidence of eyewitness identifications as well as the reliability of confession evidence.

PROTECTING FAMILIES, CHILDREN, AND PATIENTS

Here, we provide background information on the science of false memory, with special reference to problems that have arisen with families, patients, and children. During the late 1980s and early 1990s, there was a recovered memory epidemic: a confluence of very public events in which individuals claimed to have unearthed repressed memories of being sexually abused and traumatized (Loftus, 1993). Many of these individuals appeared in public, on talk shows, or told their stories in books. A plethora of repressed memories emerged, with allegations of sexual abuse and participation in satanic cults and rituals, often leveled against parents and grandparents. There were public recovery experiences by celebrities. Roseanne Barr, for example, discussed repressed memories of abuse that emerged after therapeutic treatment. On the Sally Jesse Raphael talk show, she claimed to have memories of being molested by her mother at the age of 6 months. She also expressed that her parents sexually abused her two sisters, her brother, and even her own child. Roseanne's story was highly publicized through popular articles, appearing on the cover of *People* magazine (Loftus, 1993).

Psychotherapy also had a recovered memory crisis in the late 1980s and early 1990s, which resulted in some high-profile legal cases. Certain approaches to psychotherapy promoted the idea that individuals could repress memories of traumatic events, but through psychotherapeutic treatment, these memories might come flooding back. In many cases, patients later concluded that their memories were false and sued their therapists (Brainerd & Reyna, 2005). One illustration of this issue involved 19-year-old Beth Rutherford, who began counseling sessions believing she had experienced a happy childhood with loving parents. The counseling sessions focused increasingly on the sexual abuse theme and on the recovery of her supposed repressed memories of abuse. After 2½ years of counseling, Rutherford had recovered highly specific "memories" of repeated sexual abuse by her father between the ages of 7 and 14, including being raped by him with a fork and scissors (Brainerd & Reyna, 2005). Eventually she became aware that some of her memories, such as being impregnated by her father and having multiple abortions, were medically impossible. After Rutherford realized her memories were unquestionably false, her family filed suit against the counselor for malpractice and defamation, accepting a settlement of $1 million.

Rutherford was just one of many highly publicized legal cases emphasizing that psychotherapeutic treatment may implant false memories of childhood sexual abuse (see Reyna, Holliday, & Marche, 2002, for a discussion of implantation of false memories). As a result of litigation against therapists for having implanted false memories of horrific childhood experiences (Simpson, 1996), professional organizations such as the American Medical Association and the

American Psychological Association released statements that described the potential unreliability of therapeutically stimulated recovery of memories of childhood trauma, particularly childhood sexual abuse (Brainerd & Reyna, 2005).

The McMartin Preschool trial was a day care sexual abuse case of the 1980s and an example of false memory in children. Raymond Buckey, along with his mother, operated a preschool in California. Judy Johnson, the mother of a 2-year-old boy, reported to police that her son had been sexually abused by Buckey. Eventually, numerous charges involving sexual abuse and molestation were leveled against both Buckey and his mother. Raymond Buckey was arrested and a letter from the police was sent to the parents of McMartin Preschool children requesting relevant information regarding sexual abuse. The letter contained highly suggestive material, which explained specific sexual acts that were suspected to have occurred. Several months later, staff from the Children's Institute International diagnosed more than 350 children as victims of sexual abuse at the McMartin Preschool. The founder of the school and six teachers were charged with more than 100 counts of child sexual abuse. After 6 years and two criminal trials, no convictions were obtained. Buckey's mother was acquitted on all charges in the first trial and prosecutors decided, after Buckey's second trial, not to go to trial for the third time on the remaining counts. The second trial, like the first, produced a hung jury on 13 counts (*State of California v. Buckey*, 1990). Some jurors concluded that it was impossible to convict the defendants on any of the counts because the interviews during which the children were questioned about sexual abuse, which the jurors had been shown on videotape, were highly suggestive (Ceci & Bruck, 1995). The McMartin Preschool trial is an example of an instance in which prosecutions of defendants were allowed to proceed even though the statements of child witnesses contained descriptions of features of crimes that were disproved by physical evidence.

FALSE CONFESSIONS AND FALSE EYEWITNESS IDENTIFICATION

Next, we discuss criminal cases that involved false confessions and false identifications, providing additional examples for why the scientific study of false memory is so crucial to the law. In 1997, the Department of Justice conducted a study of false convictions and false eyewitness identifications. The study found that 90% of convictions involved positive identifications (which must have been false memories because the defendants were innocent, as proven by DNA and other physical evidence). Many cases involved positive identifications of the same person made by multiple witnesses (eight in one case), all based on false memories (Wells et al., 1998). Furthermore, many cases dealing with false confessions have been documented (e.g., Gudjonsson & MacKeith, 1990). Three *Chicago Tribune* reporters provided evidence of the potential scope of this phenomenon (Armstrong, Milles, & Possley, 2001) by reviewing court records of murder cases dating back to 1991. Armstrong et al. (2001) identified 247 cases in which police interviewers had obtained self-incriminating statements from defendants. Investigators went forward with prosecution, but the confessions were later judged to have been false. Judges viewed statements as being clearly false or contaminated, or the statements had failed to produce convictions because juries interpreted them as false. The 247 cases included false confessions from suspects who had been in jail when the crimes occurred, confessions that were refuted by DNA evidence, and confessions that were refuted by other physical evidence.

The real danger of false confessions is that the scientific literature shows that juries believe confessions. Psychologically, a jury cannot ignore a confession once it comes forward (Brainerd & Reyna, 2005), even if instructed to do so by a judge. Why? Juries simply believe that people will not falsely confess to something they have not done (Kassin & Sukel, 1997) and therefore think that confessions are highly reliable. Because investigators and prosecutors naturally favor presenting evidence that will convince jurors, there is a strong motivation to obtain confessions.

Not only has research confirmed that people give false confessions, it also has shown that such confessions come in three varieties. The first is a *spontaneous voluntary confession*. Highly publicized cases are infamous for stimulating voluntary false confessions. Mental illness, including delusional states, is often cited as a reason for voluntary false confessions (Kassin, 1997), but sane individuals who make false confessions sometimes claim that they were longing for attention (Wrightsman & Kassin, 1993). One such example may have occurred in the case of JonBenét Ramsey, a 6-year-old beauty pageant contestant who was found murdered in her Colorado home. An elementary school teacher, John Mark Karr, falsely confessed to killing her, but many inconsistencies between his confession and the actual crime were apparent. Karr claimed that he drugged and raped the girl before accidentally killing her, but her autopsy found no evidence of drugs, and she was strangled after being beaten. He also claimed that he picked up JonBenét from school before killing her, even though the murder took place during the Christmas holidays. Moreover, Karr's former wife said she was with him in Alabama during the time of the killing. She explained that Karr was enthralled with the Ramsey murder and spent considerable time researching the case. Eventually, Karr's confession was dismissed because DNA tests failed to link him to the crime scene.

Another type of false confession is *coerced-compliant confession*, which can result from suggestive interviewing tactics. Often, individuals make self-incriminating statements during the course of police interviews or inter-rogations and even sign written confession statements, even though they have no memory of the crimes and do not believe they committed them. The 1989 "Central Park jogger" case in New York City is an example of a false coerced-compliant confession. The victim was an investment banker who, according to accusations, had been raped and beaten by a group of African American and Hispanic youths. Police interrogations resulted in false confessions, which were later disproved by DNA tests of semen samples. Moreover, the individual who actually committed the crime later confessed, exonerating the defendants (Ryan, 1989). As a second example, Douglas Warney falsely confessed to murder and served 10 years in prison before being freed by DNA evidence (*Warney v. State of New York*, 2010). When subjected to suggestive police interrogations, Warney confessed to the murder of civil rights activist William Beason. His lawyers argued that the confession was con-taminated with memory errors and was the ranting of a man with dementia. The Warney case illustrates two key factors that are usually associated with coerced-compliant confessions: (a) strong memory suggestion in the form of false evidence that seems more reliable than memory and (b) suspects who are specifically vulnerable to memory falsification (Brainerd & Reyna, 2005; Kassin, 1997; Reyna & Brainerd, 1998).

The third form of false confession is *coerced-internalized confession*, a type that is based squarely on false memories and therefore is not usually recanted. Suspects will make self-incriminating statements in which they actually "remember" the events and crimes they think they committed, even though these statements are disproved by other evidence. A famous case involved police officer Paul Ingram (Brainerd & Reyna, 2005). Ingram was accused of raping his daughter, participating in satanic rituals, and murdering babies. His church minister pressured him to confess, while his psychologist explained to him that sexual abusers usually repress memories of their crimes. Over time, Ingram remembered committing these crimes, pleaded guilty, and was sentenced to 20 years in prison. Eventually, sociologist Robert Ofshe concluded that the confessions stemmed from memory suggestions when he found that he was able to induce Ingram to remember and confess to other crimes (Ofshe & Watters, 1994).

In addition to prosecution of the innocent, evidence that is infected with false memories can allow the guilty to go free and reoffend. This issue was recently illustrated in the case of Elizabeth Smart. Smart, a 14-year-old, was kidnapped from her bed in the middle of the night. There was no significant forensic evidence (i.e., fingerprints, DNA samples) regarding her abduction (Haberman & MacIntosh, 2003). Jean Boylan, a retired FBI forensic artist, interviewed Elizabeth's sister, volunteering to make a sketch of the man that she saw kidnap Elizabeth. Ms. Boylan emphasizes avoidance of suggestion in her work, sometimes spending many hours listening to a witness before producing a sketch. The sketch that she produced in this case strongly resembled Brian Mitchell, the actual abductor. However, the police did not believe that he was the perpetrator and focused on another suspect, Richard Ricci, based on inaccurate memory reports by various witnesses. That suspect eventually died in prison while Elizabeth Smart remained in the custody of her abductor and was victimized for more than 9 months. Fortunately, Ms. Smart was ultimately recognized while walking on the street with her abductor.

THE SCIENCE OF FALSE MEMORY

We now summarize some of the scientific concepts and findings explaining the aforementioned false memories. First, what is *false memory?* It is remembering something that did not happen as though it did. To study false memory, researchers need to know which memories are true and which are false. That is impossible with the "on the street" memories in crimes because there is no record of what actually happened. To know which memories are true and which are false, researchers take memory off the streets and into the laboratory. In the laboratory, scientists can manipulate and control variables while knowing concretely which memories are false. Participants can be exposed to staged crimes or other events, and researchers can study what circumstances cause false memories of events. Researchers can manipulate potential causes of false memory to establish true cause–effect relations. In addition, the results of laboratory research on memory have often produced seemingly counterintuitive results that violate both commonsense and legal assumptions. Such violations are almost never apparent on the streets.

Several theories are applied in understanding false memory (e.g., constructivism, schema theory, source monitoring; for a review, see Brainerd & Reyna, 2001). But well-known limitations prevent them from accounting for many modern false memory findings (Brainerd & Reyna, 2005). A more recent account of false memory is provided by fuzzy trace theory, which was developed by the second and third authors of this chapter (Reyna & Brainerd, 1995). *Fuzzy trace* is a theory of decision making and memory processing that holds that individuals are predisposed to rely on imprecise gist cognitive processing in making decisions and even in performing memory tasks. Having an option, people prefer to minimize the amount of detail they use in making a decision. Two types of memory traces can be encoded for a given memory experience: gist traces and verbatim traces. *Gist traces* maintain the meaning of the memory event. These traces reflect abstract properties and semantic representations—how one interprets an experience. *Verbatim traces* maintain the surface qualities and context of a memory, providing the specific details that people remember of a past experience, and usually fade over time. The two types of traces reinforce each other with regard to true memories. The two traces oppose each other in fomenting (gist) or suppressing (verbatim) false memory (Brainerd & Reyna, 2002).

An everyday example of the verbatim–gist distinction is the food eaten at a baseball game. An individual attends a baseball game and remembers who he was with, which teams were playing, the score, and who won. These are examples of verbatim memories. Later on, someone asks him, "Did you eat a hot dog at the game?" He thinks to himself and goes through the gist of the experience, how he feels about and understands the meaning of the event. The attendee realizes that at many baseball games, he does eat "junk food" such as hot dogs. He remembers eating junk food. As a result, he concludes he probably ate a hot dog, when in fact he ate pizza. In this situation, verbatim memory may trump his inference that he had a hot dog. Good verbatim memory suppresses false memories. However, the science also demonstrates that strong gist memories will elevate false memories, in which case the attendee is likely to say, "Sure, I probably had a hot dog."

Although gist traces cause false memories, scientific evidence shows that people rely on them extensively because, for the most part, they do not create memories that violate the facts of experience (Reyna & Brainerd, 1995, 1998). Memories that are consistent with the gist of the experience are usually true (e.g., having hot dogs at baseball games or reading menus at restaurants). Individuals also rely on gist traces because verbatim traces of the details of experiences fade rapidly and they are left with the *halo* of the experience, that is, the overall summary or feeling of the event. Gist traces are what people have left after verbatim traces fade away (i.e., become inaccessible).

An important strength of fuzzy trace theory is that it is able to predict highly counterintuitive findings about false memory, such as developmental reversals (Ceci & Bruck, 1998; Reyna & Brainerd, 1998), which violate some historical assumptions and common beliefs held in courtrooms. In court, children are often challenged as unreliable witnesses on the grounds that they are prone to false memory (Reyna, et al., 2007). Other things being equal, if there are conflicting reports from children and adults, the latter are considered more reliable. This presumption of unreliability is so prevalent that some judges have ruled it as commonsense knowledge among jurors (Brainerd et al., 2008). Fuzzy trace theory, however, predicts that some important types of false memories, based on the gist of experiences, will increase between childhood and adulthood (Reyna & Brainerd, 1998). Adults are more likely to rely on certain types of gist because meaning comprehension of experiences and the ability to connect meaning across experiences improve dramatically with development (Bjorklund, 2004).

Research has shown that the ability to connect meaning across everyday events and experiences develops slowly in children and adolescents. In an empirical demonstration of this, children, adolescents, and young adults are given materials to remember that have strong meaning connections (like a set of everyday experiences). Two prominent results are exhibited: False memory for meaning-consistent events increases with age, and sometimes the increase in false memory is bigger than the corresponding age increase in true memory (see also Reyna & Farley, 2006, for developmental increases in meaning-based illusions in judgment and decision making). The data show that some types of gist/meaning-based false memories increase as children develop into adults (Brainerd & Reyna, 2002). In some situations, false memory is much lower in children than in adults because children have not yet had the rich experience required to develop gist memory. Since 2002, these age increases in false memory have been confirmed in dozens of experiments that illustrated how memory can be more accurate in children than in adults (Brainerd, Reyna, & Ceci, 2008). The weight of scientific evidence now suggests that false memories normally increase with age when they require connecting meaning across events (Brainerd, Reyna, & Zember, 2011; Reyna, Mills, et al., 2007).

In addition to developmental reversals, several other findings about false memory run counter to the law's assumptions. In the remainder of this section, we review some key examples that concern forgetting phenomena. Legal common sense assumes that *true memory reports*, which refer to actual experiences, have more cognitive support than *false memory reports*, which refer to events that were not experienced. Some obvious predictions from this are that false memory reports should be unstable over time and true memory reports should have a stability advantage over false ones. These predictions are considered commonsense expectations in the law and are known as the *consistency principle* of testimony (Brainerd & Reyna, 2005). Judges and juries often apply this principle when weighing the credibility of evidence; that is, the consistency of memory reports over time figures prominently in their deliberations. A common assumption is that events that have been inconsistently reported are less likely to be true than those that have been reported over extended periods of time (Fisher & Cutler, 1992).

However, fuzzy trace theory predicts that false memory reports are sometimes more stable than true memory reports (Reyna & Lloyd, 1997). This prediction, known as the *false-persistence effect*, posits that false memories will have a stability advantage when (a) initial false memory reports are rooted in gist memory; (b) initial true memory reports are skewed toward verbatim memory; and (c) over time, verbatim memories become inaccessible more rapidly than gist (Brainerd & Reyna, 2005). The retrieval of verbatim traces suppresses false memory reports by deactivating the gist traces that elevate false memory. However, verbatim retrieval is more likely to occur on initial memory tests than on delayed memory tests (Brainerd, Reyna, & Brandse, 1995). Accordingly, there may be high rates of consistency between false memory on initial and delayed memory reports. That would mean less consistency over time in true reports than in false ones, which is the opposite of what the law assumes.

A second and more surprising forgetting phenomenon from the perspective of the law is *false superiority*. Common sense states that the most likely events to be reported in the court should be events based on true memories (Brainerd & Reyna, 2005). It is commonly believed that events based on true memories are more likely to be reported in the court. Specifically, true memories are likely to trump false memories. However, according to fuzzy trace theory, there are circumstances in which events that did not happen will be better remembered than events that did happen, the specific circumstances being ones in which false events provide far better fits to the gist of experience than true. Experiments have been reported that confirm this prediction (Brainerd & Reyna, 1998).

FROM RESEARCH TO TRANSLATION: LAW, PSYCHOLOGY, AND HUMAN DEVELOPMENT

In this section, we discuss examples of memory research in children and adults, as well as judgment and decision-making research and how both translate into legal practice. Translational research has the potential to drive the advancement of applied science. The challenge for researchers is to take phenomena off the streets and into the research lab, but then to take them "back to the streets," where research findings can improve practice and policy.

Memory is a key consideration in a number of fields related to human welfare, including medicine as well as the law (Reyna, 2008). In criminal investigations, as we explained earlier in this chapter, physical evidence that can be used in the courts is often lacking. Even when it is gathered, physical evidence is processed less than 50% of the time and is usually treated as an adjunct to memory reports (e.g., Horvath & Meesig, 1996). The legal evidence in criminal investigations often comes down to human memory—including eyewitness identifications, police reports, witness interviews, written narratives, suspect interrogations, trial testimony, telephone conversations, e-mails, and depositions—and to what people do with the information they have (judgment and decision making). Thus, in the law, translational research involves understanding the principles that govern what people remember about their experience and what people do with what they remember (Reyna, Mills, et al., 2007).

Many times, even physical evidence/forensic science used in legal cases is presented in memory form (i.e., expert testimony given to the jury). Witnesses' memory reports enter as legal evidence every step of the way, from the occurrence of a crime to the last witness in a trial. For the most part, then, that memory is the evidence. Errors in any of these memory reports are difficult to disprove because of the lack of tangible physical evidence (Ceci & Friedman, 2000; Dunning & Stern, 1994). Since memory is the primary evidence in the law, we must understand what causes false memories and which types of people may be vulnerable to them.

Although multiple research areas in psychology can be applied to translational research in the law, we focus primarily on the science of human memory. Translation is especially crucial in the law because, as we have seen, the science shows that many common legal assumptions are mistaken. It is important for this science to enter mainstream practice by influencing what judges and juries believe. That is because our justice systems rely squarely on the assumptions that judges and juries make in their role as triers of fact. We have previously discussed some assumptions that can lead to erroneous legal decisions because they are known to be wrong scientifically.

Translational Memory Research With Children

Memory research currently supplies the most examples of translation to the law. The study of false memory, why it happens, and to whom it happens is relevant in all legal cases, particularly criminal investigations. The role of forgetting in increasing false memory reports has been extensively demonstrated, especially in children. The translational significance of such work is high because when children are witnesses or victims of crimes, extended periods of time between when the events occur and when those memory reports are used as legal evidence may have elapsed. For example, in the United States, for common felonies such as robbery, assault, drug possession, or drug sales, an interval of several months is the minimum delay between the charging of a crime and the actual trial. In fact, delays of 1 or 2 years are not uncommon (Brainerd & Reyna, 2005). In capital cases, there may be delays of years. In addition, there are typically prolonged delays between the charging of a crime and the time when a child witness is first interviewed by the police. Sometimes children are too emotionally or physically traumatized and parents refuse interview requests for extended periods of time, or police officers are too busy to conduct interviews directly after a crime. Another reason for delays is that new evidence must be assessed. This new evidence, which could be discovered weeks, months, or years after the crime, may then direct investigators toward a particular child whose memory has not been previously probed.

This is significant for translation because research shows that delays dilute the accuracy of memory reports taken from child witnesses and victims. Children's true memory reports will decline over delays (Brainerd, 1997; Reyna & Kiernan, 1995), and their false memory reports will increase (Poole & White, 1995; Reyna & Kiernan, 1994). That makes perfect sense from the standpoint of the basic science that we have covered: If verbatim and gist traces are both available at Time 1, by Time 2 (say, 1 week later), forgetting processes will have degraded verbatim traces more than gist traces.

When it comes to child witnesses, perhaps the best-known area of translational research is *suggestive questioning*. During the 1980s, there was a significant shift in legal attitudes about what was considered appropriate questioning of children that derived from such research (Ceci & Friedman, 2000). In child sexual abuse cases, the only witnesses are normally a single child victim and a single adult perpetrator. Since the crimes do not usually leave any reliable physical evidence, the only source of evidence is usually children's memory reports. The majority of reported victims of such crimes are not adolescents or elementary school children, but preschoolers and children in the first few elementary grades (Poole & Lamb, 1998). Many times when children in this age range are questioned, the only information they can provide in response to open-ended questions is their name and age (Howe, 1991). However, these children will often provide detailed information about specific acts of abuse in response to leading questions, such as "Did Mr. Johnson touch your privates yesterday?" This type of suggestive questioning about crimes has been found to induce false memory reports in child witnesses (Ceci & Bruck, 1995), but it has been argued that children are resistant to falsification when the target memories are of traumatic events that they directly experienced. That proposal has been the subject of considerable research and has been disconfirmed (Ceci & Friedman, 2000).

Suggestive questioning of children is highly relevant to the law because in actual field interviews in cases of suspected sexual abuse, suggestive interview procedures are permissible (Ceci & Bruck, 1995). Studies of court cases (e.g., *State of California v. Buckey*, 1990) reveal that such procedures may include (a) repeating a previously answered question several times within an interview, (b) selectively reinforcing desired responses (e.g., "Yes, that's the right answer. You're doing great now"), (c) stereotyping of suspects (e.g., "Mr. Smith is a pretty bad guy"), (d) peer pressure to agree with allegations of abuse (e.g., "Your friend Sally was here today, and she told me that Mr. Smith touched her privates, too"), and (e) guided imagery (e.g., "Try to see in your head what Mr. Smith did to you. Just get a clear picture of what he did when he was touching you"). Controlled experimentation has established that such procedures are capable of producing false memory reports in adult witnesses, victims, and suspects, and it is reasonable to believe that they will have similar effects on children.

We explained earlier in this chapter that gist-based false memory reports can increase dramatically with age, which has obvious translational significance in legal cases that involve child witnesses, victims, or suspects. However, another fact of obvious translational significance in such cases is that the accuracy of verbatim-based true memory also increases with age. Thus, memory for the surface details of an event exhibit age improvements, with initial improvements during the preschool and elementary school years being greater than subsequent ones (e.g., Brainerd, 1997; Brainerd, Reyna, & Brandse, 1995; Brainerd, Stein, & Reyna, 1998; Reyna & Kiernan, 1994, 1995). This means that translational memory research confronts the law with a seeming paradox: False memories for events with strong meaning connections (such events are standard fare in legal cases) will often increase with age, but so will true memory for actual details of events.

Translational Memory Research With Adults

Memory decline during healthy aging is another area that translates to the law. Most of the research on this topic has focused on evaluating declines in true memories and determining the conditions affecting such declines (e.g., Bowles & Salthouse, 2003; Brainerd, Reyna, & Howe, 2009; Dunlosky & Salthouse, 1996; Reyna & Mills, 2007). Areas of true memory performance that exhibit significant declines have been identified and compared with areas that display little or no decline. For example, aging is known to have a large effect on the accuracy of eyewitness identifications, particularly facial memory (Bartlett & Fulton, 1991; Bartlett & Leslie, 1985, 1986). Research has focused on applications to naturalistic criminal identification situations (e.g., subjects respond to photo spreads after observing a sequence of events in which a crime was committed). It is well established that older adults perform worse than younger adults at correctly rejecting mug shots of innocent people.

In that connection, Bartlett reported several findings that emphasize an increased reliance on gist processing over verbatim processing in eyewitness identification during later adulthood, resulting in decreased accuracy (Bartlett & Fulton, 1991). There are two theoretical explanations for this shift in processing: verbatim deficit and gist preference. The *verbatim-deficit* conjecture claims that elderly adults fail to store verbatim traces of target materials (Brainerd & Reyna, 2005). Even when verbatim traces are stored, they may fade at a more rapid rate than in younger adults. As a result, older adults have no choice but to rely on gist processing. On the other hand, the *gist-preference* conjecture claims that elderly adults naturally prefer to retrieve gist memories over verbatim traces—they tend to focus on meaning content even when verbatim traces are available (Kouststaal et al., 2003).

The accuracy and confidence of adults' eyewitness identifications are especially clear examples of how memory research translates into legal practice. Eyewitness identifications are central to some of the most serious types of crimes (e.g., armed robbery, drug sales, rape, shootings), and such cases often cannot be prosecuted without positive identification of suspects by victims or other witnesses. Haber and Haber (2004) reviewed more than 500 research articles to understand the accuracy of eyewitness identifications under good conditions, a type of information that is essential for juries in interpreting eyewitness identification evidence in trials. These researchers selected 37 articles reporting a total of 48 experiments in which eyewitness identifications were made under good conditions (e.g., culprits could be clearly seen, identifications were made within a reasonable time after observation, identifications were made using lineups or photo spreads with four or more choices).

In the eyewitness identification tests used in these experiments, the culprit was either present or absent. When the culprit is absent from the test stimuli, two responses are possible: a wrong choice (false memory response) and no choice (true memory response). When the culprit is present in the test stimuli, three responses are possible: a wrong choice (false memory response), a correct choice (true memory response), and no choice (a no-memory response). In legal investigations, the culprit-absent data are more important because defendants usually are under a constitutional assumption of innocence. Thus, if an eyewitness has identified a defendant, the defense's position will normally be that the actual culprit was not present in the photo spread or lineup that was used, and that the identification is therefore false (Brainerd & Reyna, 2005). Results from Haber and Haber's (2004) baseline reliability research supported the defense position. When the culprit was absent, subjects falsely identified someone innocent 57% of the time. In contrast, the prosecution position will be that the culprit was present in the test stimuli, that the defendant is the culprit, and that the identification is correct. This position is not supported by the research findings (Haber & Haber, 2004). When the culprit was present, subjects correctly identified that person only 51% of the time, and they falsely identified another innocent person 27% of the time. The research therefore suggests that the overall accuracy level is analogous to flipping a coin. In addition, normal eyewitness identifications usually do not have the favorable conditions of the "best case" experiments that Haber and Haber selected. Clearly, the extensive research in their review severely questions the reliability of real-life eyewitness identifications.

This point is further illustrated by defendants who were convicted at trial with positive eyewitness identifications but later exonerated. After the introduction of DNA evidence, the National Institute of Justice released a study of

28 cases in which defendants had been convicted on the basis of eyewitness identifications and exonerated after serving extended time in prison (Connors, Lundregan, Miller, & McEwan, 1996). In some cases, multiple positive identifications of one defendant were made. Over the course of several years, researchers (e.g., Kassin, 1998; Wells et al., 1998) have concluded that false identifications lead to more wrongful convictions than all other causes combined.

Although the high error rates in eyewitness identifications are troubling and perplexing to the law, they are readily explained via fuzzy trace theory's distinction between verbatim and gist memory traces (Brainerd & Reyna, 2005). Recognizing the face of a culprit who was observed at a crime scene is a verbatim memory task and a rather difficult one. However, we know that verbatim memory traces become rapidly inaccessible over time, leaving more stable gist traces as the basis for identification. We also know that gist traces can lead to false identification because innocent suspects often fit the gist of actual culprits (e.g., are the same gender, age, ethnicity, and body build). As time passes from the crime to the trial, gist traces may be the only memory support left for eyewitness identifications (e.g., witnesses only remember that the suspect was a young, thin, Hispanic male).

The memory effects of psychotherapy and counseling are a final topic in memory research whose translational significance is high for the law. We have seen that in the 1980s and 1990s, potential memory distortions that arose from psychotherapy were subjects of both civil and criminal proceedings. The ongoing problem for the law is that people who are involved in legal cases, witnesses and victims in particular, often receive psychotherapy or counseling before trial. In fact, people are often sent to therapy by court order. This is particularly true in serious crimes (e.g., rape, death, injury of loved ones). Naturally, the focus of the psychotherapy or counseling is on alleviating the effects of the traumas that are by-products of crimes. Unfortunately, it is well-known scientifically that psychotherapeutic techniques that are often used to achieve that goal can distort memory accuracy for the traumatic experiences (Brainerd & Reyna, 2005).

Afterword on Translational Research in Judgment and Decision Making

Up to this point, we have focused on false memory research as it bears on the task of witnesses, which is to faithfully report the facts as they remember them. However, there are other important players in trials—prosecutors, defense attorneys, judges, and juries. Their tasks involve making judgments and decisions, not verbatim memory reports. Juries, in particular, are charged with judging the credibility of the evidence that is presented, and good performance means convicting the guilty and acquitting the innocent, not simply remembering the facts of a case. Gist, which we have seen is a cause of false memory in witnesses, can be the basis of superior judgment and decision making (Reyna, 2008).

Adults base their reasoning on gist representations of information whenever possible. As individuals develop and gain experience, a preference evolves for processing gist, and intuitive gist-based reasoning increases relative to analytical verbatim-based reasoning (Reyna, 2004). In decisions that involve risk (e.g., drinking and driving, unprotected sex), this can lead to correct risk-avoidance decisions (Reyna & Farley, 2006). However, when reasoners rely on verbatim memory and analytical reasoning (e.g., calculating the odds), they may choose the riskier option. For example, in a game of Russian roulette, people should rely on the gist representation, "You could die!" over the verbatim representation, which would involve calculating the odds. The odds are against a fatal outcome, but it is still a bad idea.

A final point about the translational value of judgment and decision making research is that it is particularly important to understand the changes in gist- versus verbatim-based reasoning in adolescence and early adulthood. Young adults commit most crimes, and these acts often originate in risky behaviors that are first practiced during adolescence. The majority of crimes committed by young adults occur either when they are impaired by alcohol or drugs or are stealing to get funds to acquire alcohol or drugs. Studies show that the use of alcohol, drugs, and cigarettes is initiated in youth (Reyna & Farley, 2006). To deal with such cases, the law must understand basic scientific findings on risky behavior in adolescence, findings showing that the simple gists that adults use to make decisions about risk ("I could die") are not yet in frequent use among teens.

CONCLUSION

In this chapter, we surveyed some of the translational possibilities of false memory research from the perspective of the law. We described the recovered memory crisis of the late 1980s and early 1990s, and the realization that people could "recover" false memories of horrific experiences provided a strong stimulus to scientific study of false memory. We then sketched historical assumptions that the law makes about human memory that are not supported by research findings, even though the assumptions have strong commonsense support (e.g., that true events are more likely to be reported than false ones, that children's reports are always more distorted than those of adults). We also examined how these erroneous assumptions, together with other features of criminal processing, can lead to false confessions, false accusations, and false convictions.

We also described how memory research has generated theoretical principles, such as the verbatim–gist distinction, that are of high translational value in the law. It has also generated research findings on the specific memory phenomena that are of high translational value (e.g., the effects of suggestive questioning, the effects of delay, the accuracy of eyewitness identifications). Ideally, in the future, researchers will have a much more extensive catalogue of experimental findings on the accuracy of theoretical predictions about key memory phenomena in the law. Finally, we briefly illustrated the translational value of judgment and decision-making research in the law.

The ultimate objective of such translational research is to ensure that scientific findings and empirically validated theoretical principles are integrated into the courtroom and other areas of legal proceedings. This has already begun and can be seen in multiple scenarios related to the courtroom.

Michael Lamb and associates at the Eunice Kennedy Shriver National Institute of Child Health and Human Development (NICHD) developed a protocol for the forensic investigative interviewing of children. After the McMartin and other infamous child abuse cases, the need for extensive laboratory and field research in regard to obtaining information from children was apparent (Brainerd & Reyna, 2005). The NICHD protocol consists of a series of steps that interviewers are instructed to follow. The structure of the memory questions corresponds with what research has highlighted regarding the nature of questions that produce true versus false memories.

Another example of research implemented professionally in the courtroom is the eyewitness identification guidelines published by the Department of Justice in 1999. After realizing that eyewitness identifications were highly error prone, many leading scientists in memory and eyewitness identification gathered together and produced a manual of procedures for the police to follow. The guidelines consist of recommendations for mug books, lineups and photo spreads. These procedures prevent eyewitness identifications from being contaminated in any obvious ways (Brainerd & Reyna, 2005).

If there is an increase in legal knowledge of false memory and how it works, investigations and trials are bound to reflect the actual events of legal cases more accurately because judges, juries, and legal professionals will be relying more on science and less on mistaken assumptions. The result will be a justice system that is more just.

REFERENCES

Armstrong, K., Milles, S., & Possley, M. (2001, December 16). Coercive and illegal tactics torpedo scores of Cook County murder cases. *Chicago Tribune*. Retrieved from http://www.chicagotribune.com/news/watchdog/chi-011216confession, 0,1748927.story

Bartlett, J. C., & Fulton, A. (1991). Familiarity and recognition of faces in old age. *Memory & Cognition, 19,* 229–238. doi:10.3758/BF03211147

Bartlett, J. C., & Leslie, J. E. (1985). Age-differences in memory for faces vs. views of faces. *Bulletin of the Psychonomic Society, 23,* 285.

Bartlett, J. C., & Leslie, J. E. (1986). Aging and memory for faces versus single views of faces. *Memory & Cognition, 14,* 371–381. doi:10.3758/BF03197012

Bjorklund, D. F. (2004). *Children's thinking: Cognitive development and individual differences.* Belmont, CA: Wadsworth.

Bowles, R. P., & Salthouse, T. A. (2003). Assessing the age-related effects of proactive interference on working memory tasks using the Rasch model. *Psychology and Aging, 18,* 608–615. doi:10.1037/0882-7974.18.3.608

Brainerd, C. J. (1997). Development of forgetting, with implications for memory suggestibility. In N. L. Stein, P. A. Ornstein, B. Tversky, & C. J. Brainerd (Eds.), *Memory for everyday and emotional events* (pp. 209–235). Hillsdale, NJ: Erlbaum.

Brainerd, C. J., & Reyna, V. F. (1998). When things that were never experienced are easier to "remember" than things that were. *Psychological Science, 9,* 484–489. doi:10.1111/1467-9280.00089

Brainerd, C. J., & Reyna, V. F. (2001). Fuzzy-trace theory: Dual-processes in reasoning, memory, and cognitive neuroscience. *Advances in Child Development and Behavior, 28,* 41–100.

Brainerd, C. J., & Reyna, V. F. (2002). Fuzzy-trace theory and false memory. *Current Directions in Psychological Science, 11,* 164–169. doi:10.1111/1467-8721.00192

Brainerd, C. J., & Reyna, V. F. (2005). *The science of false memory.* New York, NY: Oxford University Press. doi:10.1093/acprof:oso/9780195154054.001.0001

Brainerd, C. J., Reyna, V. F., & Brandse, E. (1995). Are children's false memories more persistent than their true memories? *Psychological Science, 6,* 359–364. doi:10.1111/j.1467-9280.1995.tb00526.x

Brainerd, C. J., Reyna, V. F., & Ceci, S. J. (2008). Developmental reversals in false memory: A review of data and theory. *Psychological Bulletin, 134,* 343–382. doi:10.1037/0033-2909.134.3.343

Brainerd, C. J., Reyna, V. F., & Howe, M. L. (2009). Trichotomous processes in early memory development, aging, and neurocognitive impairment: A unified theory. *Psychological Review, 116,* 783–832. doi:10.1037/a0016963

Brainerd, C. J., Stein, L. M., & Reyna, V. F. (1998). On the development of conscious and unconscious memory. *Developmental Psychology, 34,* 342–357. doi:10.1037/0012-1649.34.2.342

Ceci, S. J., & Bruck, M. (1995). *Jeopardy in the courtroom.* Washington, DC: American Psychological Association. doi:10.1037/10180-000

Ceci, S. J., & Bruck, M. (1998). The ontogeny and durability of true and false memories: A fuzzy trace account. *Journal of Experimental Child Psychology, 71,* 165–169. doi:10.1006/jecp.1998.2468

Ceci, S. J., & Friedman, R. D. (2000). The suggestibility of children: Scientific research and legal implications. *Cornell Law Review, 86*, 33–108.

Connors, E., Lundregan, T., Miller, N., & McEwan, T. (1996). *Convicted by juries, exonerated by science: Case studies in the use of DNA evidence to establish innocence after trial*. Alexandria, VA: National Institute of Justice.

Dunlosky, J., & Salthouse, T. A. (1996). A decomposition of age-related differences in multitrial free recall. *Aging, Neuropsychology, and Cognition, 3*(1), 2–14. doi:10.1080/13825589608256608

Dunning, D., & Stern, L. B. (1994). Distinguishing accurate from inaccurate eyewitness identifications via inquiries about decision processes. *Journal of Personality and Social Psychology, 67*, 818–835. doi:10.1037/0022-3514.67.5.818

Fisher, R. P., & Cutler, B. L. (1992, September). *The relation between consistency and accuracy of eyewitness testimony*. Paper presented at the Third European Conference on Law and Psychology, Oxford, England.

Gudjonsson, G. H., & MacKeith, J. A. C. (1990). A proven case of false confession: Psychological aspects of the coerced-compliant type. *Medicine, Science, and the Law, 30*, 329–335.

Haber, R. N., & Haber, C. (2004). *A meta-analysis of research on eyewitness line-up accuracy*. Unpublished manuscript.

Haberman, M., & MacIntosh, J. (2003). *Held captive: The kidnapping and rescue of Elizabeth Smart*. New York, NY: Avon Books.

Horvath, F., & Meesig, R. (1996). The criminal investigation process and the role of forensic evidence: A review of empirical findings. *Journal of Forensic Sciences, 41*, 133–140. doi: 10.1520/JFS14032J

Horvath, F., & Meesig, R. (1998). A content analysis of textbooks on criminal investigation: An evaluative comparison to empirical research findings in the investigative process and the role of forensic evidence. *Journal of Forensic Sciences, 43*, 133–140.

Howe, M. L. (1991). Misleading children's story recall: Forgetting and reminiscence of the facts. *Developmental Psychology, 27*, 746–762. doi:10.1037/0012-1649.27.5.746

Kassin, S. M. (1997). The psychology of confession evidence. *American Psychologist, 52*, 221–233. doi:10.1037/0003-066X.52.3.221

Kassin, S. M. (1998). Eyewitness identification procedures: The fifth rule. *Law and Human Behavior, 22*, 649–653. doi:10.1023/A:1025702722645

Kassin, S. M., & Sukel, H. (1997). Coerced confessions and the jury: An experimental test of the "harmless error" rule. *Law and Human Behavior, 21*, 27–46. doi:10.1023/A:1024814009769

Kouststaal, W., Reddy, C., Jackson, E. M., Prince, S., Cendan, D. L., & Schacter, D. L. (2003). False recognition of abstract versus common objects in older and younger adults: Testing the semantic categorization account. *Journal of Experimental Psychology: Learning, Memory, and Cognition, 29*, 499–510. doi:10.1037/0278-7393.29.4.499

Loftus, E. F. (1993). The reality of repressed memories. *American Psychologist, 48*, 518–537. doi:10.1037/0003-066X.48.5.518

Ofshe, R., & Watters, E. (1994). *Making monsters: False memories, psychotherapy, and sexual hysteria*. New York, NY: Scribner.

Poole, D. A., & Lamb, M. E. (1998). *Investigative interviews of children*. Washington, DC: American Psychological Association.

Poole, D. A., & White, L. T. (1995). Tell me again and again: Stability and change in the repeated testimonies of children and adults. In M. Zaragoza, J. R. Graham, G. N. N. Hall, R. Hirschman, & Y. S. Ben-Porath (Eds.), *Memory, suggestibility, and eyewitness testimony in children and adults* (pp. 24–43). Thousand Oaks, CA: Sage.

Reyna, V. F. (2004). How people make decisions that involve risk: A dual-processes approach. *Current Directions in Psychological Science, 13*, 60–66. doi:10.1111/j.0963-7214.2004.00275.x

Reyna, V. F. (2008). A theory of medical decision making and health: Fuzzy-trace theory. *Medical Decision Making, 28*, 850–865. doi:10.1177/0272989X08327066

Reyna, V. F., & Brainerd, C. J. (1995). Fuzzy-trace theory: An interim synthesis. *Learning and Individual Differences, 7*, 1–75. doi:10.1016/1041-6080(95)90031-4

Reyna, V. F., & Brainerd, C. J. (1998). Fuzzy-trace theory and false memory: New frontiers. *Journal of Experimental Child Psychology, 71*, 194–209. doi:10.1006/jecp.1998.2472

Reyna, V. F., & Farley, F. (2006). Risk and rationality in adolescent decision making: Implications for theory, practice, and public policy. *Psychological Science in the Public Interest, 7*, 1–44.

Reyna, V. F., Holliday, R. E., & Marche, T. (2002). Explaining the development of false memories. *Developmental Review, 22*, 436–489. doi:10.1016/S0273-2297(02)00003-5

Reyna, V. F., & Kiernan, B. (1994). The development of gist versus verbatim memory in sentence recognition: Effects of lexical familiarity, semantic content, encoding instructions, and retention interval. *Developmental Psychology, 30*, 178–191. doi:10.1037/0012-1649.30.2.178

Reyna, V. F., & Kiernan, B. (1995). Children's memory and interpretation of psychological metaphors. *Metaphor and Symbolic Activity, 10*, 309–331. doi:10.1207/s15327868ms1004_5

Reyna, V. F., & Lloyd, F. (1997). Theories of false memory in children and adults. *Learning and Individual Differences, 9*, 95–123. doi:10.1016/S1041-6080(97)90002-9

Reyna, V. F., & Mills, B. A. (2007). Interference processes in fuzzy-trace theory: Aging, Alzheimer's disease, and development. In C. MacLeod & D. Gorfein (Eds.), *Inhibition in cognition* (pp. 185–210). Washington, DC: American Psychological Association. doi:10.1037/11587-010

Reyna, V. F., Mills, B. A., Estrada, S., & Brainerd, C. J. (2007). False memory in children: Data, theory, and legal implications. In M. P. Toglia, J. D. Read, D. F. Ross, & R. C. L. Lindsay (Eds.), *The handbook of eyewitness psychology: Memory for events* (pp. 473–510). Mahwah, NJ: Erlbaum.

Ryan, N. (1989). *Affirmation in response to vacate judgment of conviction, indictment no. 4762/89.* New York, NY: Manhattan District Attorney's Office. Retrieved from http://www.ManhattanDA.org

Simpson, P. (1996). *Second thoughts: Understanding the false memory crisis and how it could affect you.* Nashville, TN: Thomas Nelson.

State of California v. Buckey. (1990). Superior Court, Los Angeles County, CA.

Warney v. State of New York (2010). Court of Appeals, Appellate Division, NY.

Wells, G. L., Small, M., Penrod, S., Malpass, R. S., Fulero, S. M., & Brimacombe, C. A. E. (1998). Eyewitness identification procedures: Recommendations for lineups and photospreads. *Law and Human Behavior, 22,* 603–647. doi:10.1023/A:1025750605807

Wrightsman, L. S., & Kassin, S. M. (1993). *Confessions in the courtroom.* Newbury Park, CA: Sage.

8

COMMUNITY–RESEARCHER PARTNERSHIPS IN AGING: THE CORNELL INSTITUTE FOR TRANSLATIONAL RESEARCH ON AGING

ELAINE WETHINGTON, KARL PILLEMER, AND RHODA MEADOR

The Cornell Institute for Translational Research on Aging (CITRA) is a sustainable community–researcher partnership in New York City that facilitates rigorous, scientific applied research on aging. It matches researchers from Cornell University with frontline staff and directors from agencies and centers that provide services to older people living in New York City. Through this process, CITRA facilitates T2 and T3 research (see Introduction, this volume) by translating scientific research into programs to improve public health

Acknowledgments: This research was funded by Edward R. Roybal Center grants (1 P30 AG022845, Karl Pillemer and Mark S. Lachs, Principal Investigators; 2 P30 AG022845, M. Carrington Reid and Karl Pillemer, Principal Investigators) from the National Institute on Aging and by a RAND/Hartford Foundation Interdisciplinary Geriatric Research Centers Initiative grant (M. Carrington Reid, Christopher S. Murtaugh, and Elaine Wethington, Principal Investigators). We are grateful to members of the Cornell Institute for Translational Research on Aging (CITRA) Community Advisory Committee for productive collaboration in developing and implementing CITRA partnership activities; to Igal Jellinek of the New York City Council of Senior Centers and Services in New York City for facilitating connections between CITRA and more than 250 aging service organizations in New York City; to Cary Reid, Risa Breckman, and Myra Sabir for their contributions to program development, community outreach, and dissemination; and to Leslie Schultz and Carrie Chalmers for their logistical support. The first author also thanks Harold Pincus, Martha Bruce, and Carla Boutin-Foster for their many contributions to refining her thinking about translational research in the social and behavioral sciences.

(Drolet & Lorenzi, 2011; Khoury et al., 2007; Westfall, Mold, & Fagnan, 2007). CITRA applies translational methods in gerontology to health and social service settings where there are critical needs for translation of evidence-based practice (National Council on Aging, 2006; Pillemer, Czaja, Schulz, & Stahl, 2003; Pillemer, Suitor, & Wethington, 2003).

The development of CITRA from 2003 through 2009 was funded by a grant from the Edward R. Roybal Center for Translational Research on Aging (hereafter referred to as the "Roybal Center") of the National Institute on Aging (1 P30 AG022845). In 2009, an additional Roybal Center grant renewed funding for the community–researcher partnership.

This chapter describes the 6-year period during which CITRA was developed (2003–2009), including the steps taken to create innovative programs and to achieve more rapid translation of social science findings into interventions and programs for older people. It describes achievements of the program as well as concerns that could not be addressed because of limited time and staff. Finally, the chapter discusses lessons learned, especially in regard to forming and maintaining productive community–researcher partnerships in the field.

Throughout this chapter, the pronoun *we* refers to CITRA researchers and staff at Cornell University.

BRIEF OVERVIEW OF CITRA

From 2003 through 2009, the CITRA partnership combined the resources and networks of two distinct groups: (a) a consortium of researchers and faculty mentees across three campuses of Cornell University—the Ithaca campus (where social and behavioral scientists are located), the Weill Cornell Medical College in New York City (with its medical school, research facilities, and health education programs), and the Weill Psychiatric Research Institute in Westchester, New York; and (b) a network of community agencies serving older adults in New York City. CITRA's primary community collaborator was the New York City Council of Senior Centers and Services (CSCS), a citywide organization that coordinates the activities of senior centers and other member agencies throughout the five boroughs of New York City and thus represents the city as a whole. Between 2003 and 2009, CSCS included more than 250 senior centers and other agencies in virtually all New York City neighborhoods and served more than 300,000 older adults.

CITRA's major mission was to create (and is now to maintain) a community–agency network that is "research ready." Senior centers and other agencies were surveyed in the first year of the project and expressed their strong willingness to collaborate on research projects. Individual contacts were also made with larger institutions serving the needs of older New Yorkers, such as the New York City Department for the Aging (DFTA), coalitions of service agencies supported by Catholic and Jewish charitable organizations, senior housing corporations, foundations, and private social service agencies. A Community Advisory Committee (CAC) consisting of 30 agency directors and community leaders promoted and facilitated the creation of agency–researcher partnerships for specific projects.

DEVELOPMENT OF CITRA

CITRA evolved from preexisting, but smaller scale, project-specific collaborations between social gerontologists in Ithaca and geriatric researchers at Weill Cornell Medical College. These collaborations were funded in 1993 by a Roybal Center grant. During the first 10 years, the Roybal Center program at Cornell was funded as a conventional National Institutes of Health (NIH) program, with investigators pursuing independent projects connected by the theme of social integration in the second half of life (Pillemer, Moen, Wethington, & Glasgow, 2000). The program had a strong methodological core and a small pilot studies program to develop new faculty investigators (both of which were later strengthened for CITRA).

In 2003, the National Institute on Aging reestablished the Roybal Center program as CITRA—a methodological and research development infrastructure with a core mission of emphasizing and encouraging rapid translation of basic social science research into projects that would have an impact on the health and well-being of older people. Whereas the previous program consisted of linked independent R01-style research projects, CITRA used a P30 funding mechanism to promote the development of innovative translational approaches to practical problems of aging by funding small pilot projects, core educational activities, and sharing of methodological expertise among an interdisciplinary group of investigators. CITRA investigators built on the theme of the first 10 years of the Roybal Center program, which was social integration in later life (Pillemer et al., 2000).

Although not published when CITRA was first funded in 2003, the following quotation from a report by the NIH Office of Behavioral and Social Science Research (OBSSR) epitomizes the approach we took:

> To maximize the population impact of scientific discovery . . . research products need to be translated into practical applications that are then implemented effectively and efficiently in real-world settings, disseminated broadly to all stakeholders, adopted by organizations and institutions, and maintained through policies. (OBSSR, 2007, p. 17)

Through CITRA, we set the goal of developing research programs in New York City that are "informed by the needs of end-users" (OBSSR, 2007, p. 17) and community practitioners. We did this by developing an innovative seven-step translational research model to facilitate stakeholder participation in research while building the capacity of the community to collaborate in research with multi- and interdisciplinary teams of social and medical scientists:

1. creating a research-ready network of service agencies,
2. assessing community-based needs to establish a shared research agenda for the program,
3. developing a pool of investigators who are available and willing to collaborate with service agencies,
4. developing a pilot studies program to connect investigators to research opportunities involving community agencies,
5. developing and training investigators,
6. facilitating researcher–community partner interaction through educational events, and
7. engaging researchers and practitioners on critical issues related to aging using a research-to-practice consensus workshop model.

Through CITRA activities and collaborative problem solving with community partners, we became engaged in training investigators interested in translational research (Wethington et al., 2007), as well as conducting programs to involve community practitioners in the research development process (Sabir et al., 2006). Educational and other events were conducted to enhance "research readiness" and build capacity for collaboration in community settings (Wethington & Pillemer, 2007). The need to develop more formal methods to bridge the valleys between different parts of the translational continuum and to document those methods motivated us to begin to investigate the connections between our own efforts and those of other research scientists engaged in research translation.

In Years 1 and 2, we undertook a detailed needs assessment in the community and developed infrastructure for community-based research partnerships. In Year 3, we continued but expanded these activities, recruiting more community partners, consulting with subcommittees to develop ideas for increasing the effectiveness of the collaborations, and hosting educational and policy development conferences with partners. In addition, we strengthened our efforts to develop "translational" investigators, specifically refining our pilot studies program to develop partnerships between community agencies and researchers. We also adapted the model of the research consensus workshop to engage practitioners and researchers in two-way, equitable dialogue on research priorities for CITRA. We then moved toward evaluating partnership activities and publication and other dissemination of the methods we developed to bridge the gap between science and practice in gerontology. A number of proposals related to CITRA's work were submitted or funded, and new investigators were brought into the activities of the center. The Roybal Center grant was renewed in 2009, focused on chronic pain, and developed from a successful community–researcher partnership first funded by the pilot studies program.

A description of the seven components of the CITRA model follows.

CREATION OF A RESEARCH-READY NETWORK

The first and most important goal for CITRA was to develop strong relationships with community agencies and organizations in New York City. In the first year, we focused on ways to engage agencies serving older people in New York City as partners in intervention and applied research, using partnership principles from participatory research methods (Israel, Schulz, Parker, & Becker, 1998; Jones & Wells, 2007) that emphasized equitable sharing of ideas and research priorities through interaction. We operationalized community participatory research as systematic research undertaken in collaboration with stakeholders who represented community interests, were affected by the issue being examined, or were decision makers who could implement and adopt findings from the research and put them into practice. The principles we brought to partnership development were that (a) the needs of both groups would be recognized, (b) the researchers could find a hospitable environment in which to conduct research in community settings, and (c) the agencies could have an active role in creating research projects relevant to their needs. To carry out these partnership principles, we built a core partnership staff, recruited a community advisory committee, and organized face-to-face meetings to encourage community interest.

Planning was important even in initial stages because of the pace at which we hoped to establish a working partnership that would be primed for collaboration during the first 18 months of CITRA. The initial proposal to the National Institute on Aging outlined the steps we would follow to develop the partnership. A key factor leading to the success of the proposal was forging an alliance with a preexisting network of services for older people, the CSCS. More than 250 senior centers and frontline service agencies are linked to CSCS, representing all neighborhoods in the five boroughs of New York City. In addition, CSCS provided linkages to DFTA, which oversees services for older people. Through DFTA and our academic connections, we linked to services such as health care, mental health, home-delivered meal programs, adult protective services, the visiting nurse service, housing agencies, and residential living centers.

The Ithaca-based staff of CITRA included a director of dissemination, whose primary responsibility was to develop relationships with service agencies in New York, educational workshops on topics (e.g., new models for managing senior center services) requested by those agencies, and a regular newsletter. The director of dissemination was an expert on conducting intervention research in assisted living and other residential settings, with a long history of partnership development through Cornell Cooperative Extension and other statewide outreach programs. A director of partnership development based in New York City, with years of experience in applied health and health services research at Weill Cornell Medical College, was also available to researchers seeking to partner with community agencies. New York City organizational and communication tasks were subcontracted to CSCS. Graduate students and postdoctoral researchers in Ithaca provided support to partnership development programs, including writing scientific literature reviews and organizing events. Another partner of increasing importance over time was Cornell Cooperative Extension in New York City, which had preexisting relationships with many service agencies throughout New York and with the NIH-funded Weill Cornell Medical College Clinical and Translational Science Center, established in 2007 while CITRA was extant.

Another key step was the establishment and development of the CAC. Members of the CAC included 30 individuals broadly representing New York City service agencies for older people in areas such as mental health, senior center management, case management, frontline worker training, and long-term care. To increase our impact on local policymakers (see Minkler & Wallerstein, 2003), the CAC also included representatives from private and public groups who were involved in long-term program development. The CAC was planned with three subcommittees (Steering, Pilot Studies, and Dissemination), each meeting several times a year via phone conference or in person. Through CITRA's subcommittee structure, we solicited advice about fund-raising opportunities, emerging topics for research for intervention, topics for agency education, dissemination strategies, and direction of the pilot studies program. The CAC thus provided critical guidance for developing and defining research priority areas for the pilot studies program, methods for disseminating research information to the wider community, methods for building community agency capacity to partner with researchers, and identification of policy initiatives toward which CITRA could contribute.

COMMUNITY-BASED NEEDS ASSESSMENT

Within 2 months of the award (fall 2003), CITRA and CSCS collaborated to map out the range of issues facing senior service providers over the next 10 to 15 years in New York City. The purpose was to set priorities to direct the CITRA pilot studies program and other grant proposals. This joint effort yielded a number of important insights into the general issues facing older people in the future as well as a list of priorities for New York City.

To develop a list of priorities, we used the concept mapping method, a mixed-methods planning and evaluation procedure that combines frequently used group discussion techniques (e.g., focus groups, brainstorming) with multivariate statistical analysis and mapping techniques (Trochim & Kane, 2005). Concept mapping has been used for a large number of planning exercises and goal-setting projects, including setting the research agenda for social and behavioral sciences for NIH (OBSSR, 2007). It results in a series of descriptive maps in which the relative value and relationships among priorities identified by stakeholders are visualized. At each stage of the process, participants are actively involved in generating the priorities and labeling and interpreting the initial findings.

CSCS provided support for starting this initiative by asking New York City agency directors, workers, and senior advocates attending its annual conference to list five to 10 ideas about the future needs of aging New Yorkers. This request generated about 250 returned questionnaires, which yielded 1,512 individual statements for analysis. CITRA investigators and their students examined the statements for duplication, clarity, and relevance and reduced the list to a set of 95 unique ideas. The investigators then selected leaders and members of CSCS and research experts in gerontology and geriatrics to sort these 95 ideas into categories and to rate each of the ideas in relationship to "importance for older people" and "feasibility to execute." The preliminary analysis identified the following 13 clusters of activities: capacity of community services, economic security, communication, impairments, caregiving, housing, access to benefits, economic security, mental health and special needs, transportation, attitudes toward aging, workforce diversity and training, and engaged lifestyle (social integration). CITRA then called a group meeting in New York City for CSCS leaders, CITRA investigators, and several potential researchers. This group discussed the methods used to generate the list, critiqued the content of the initial clusters of activities generated by the concept mapping, and approved dissemination of the 13 priorities to agency and researcher communities through CSCS and the CITRA website.

DEVELOPMENT OF A POOL OF POTENTIAL INVESTIGATORS

Developing investigators committed to translational research on aging based in community partnerships was at the center of CITRA's mission and, as we learned throughout the life of CITRA, one of the most necessary steps for ensuring the success of the research partnerships. Considerable evidence shows that the lack of researchers trained in translational methods

(Israel et al., 1998) and partnership research involving communities (Horowitz, Robinson, & Seifer, 2009) is a significant barrier to conducting such research. In the first year, we scanned available lists of researcher expertise for researchers with interests in aging or community research at the three collaborating sites. On the basis of our analysis of available research expertise and what we knew about barriers to engaging in translational research, we developed advertising and programming material for CITRA funding opportunities, intended to help overcome some of the barriers that we felt prevented the engagement of researchers with community agencies.

The scan of research expertise resulted in a list of more than 70 potential Cornell investigators. These investigators were viewed as the potential pool of collaborators; they represented a wide variety of disciplines across the Cornell campuses. Members of this group were invited to become CITRA affiliates, and most agreed, with many recommending other people we should try to contact. Members of the affiliate group, their departments, and existing lists of researchers interested in life course, health, and aging issues were e-mailed regular updates describing CITRA's ongoing program activities and the pilot studies request for applications (described more fully below). The investigators hosted meetings throughout the year to inform the affiliates about current CITRA research activities and provide the opportunity to learn more about the benefits of participation. The database of investigators was continuously updated with current information about affiliates, including evolving research interests. When interested agencies approached CITRA with an idea for working with a Cornell partner, we called upon members of the affiliates list to attempt to make a match for a project. Conversely, when affiliates approached us to ask about opportunities to collaborate, we helped make a match with the director of a community agency.

Next, in close collaboration with our community partners, we developed a mentored pilot studies program to promote community–researcher partnerships (described more fully below) and to educate researchers about translational research methods and the benefits of community partnerships. In developing continuing education for interested investigators, we established a work-in-progress seminar that provided an opportunity for presubmission feedback for proposal and research papers, inviting participants from the affiliate list of relevant researchers. The seminar took place once a month and connected researchers in Ithaca and New York City via videoconference. Community collaborators also took part in some of the monthly seminars.

These activities helped us to identify and target a number of barriers to engaging researchers with service agencies in collaborative research in the Cornell context. We learned of barriers on both sides. The major barriers for researchers were opportunity costs, the lack of knowledge about how to contact and work with community agencies, and concern about the amount of time necessary to create and maintain partnerships with community agencies (closely related to the concern about opportunity costs). For community collaborators, the major barriers were lack of time and staff to make connections with researchers, lack of familiarity with the research process, and few existing connections to research centers.

We attempted to address these concerns by developing an infrastructure to lessen the perceived burden on investigators and agencies. We applied social network principles to connect the separate nodes of researcher and community practitioner networks, with CITRA core staff serving as the connectors. For example, we learned that agencies are enthusiastic about collaborating with researchers if there is support to promote and sustain these activities beyond the project. Thus, important roles for CITRA were to educate investigators about the expectations of community agencies for collaboration and to mentor investigators in the partnership process (Wethington et al., 2007). This type of investigator development addressed a central component of CITRA's goal of forging successful relationships with community agencies and organizations and providing the basis for sustaining them in future through recognition of mutual benefit.

DEVELOPMENT OF A PILOT STUDIES PROGRAM

The aim of the pilot studies program was to fund and develop new investigators who would benefit from the partnership for intervention and applied research we created with service agencies in New York City. The pilot studies program funded 21 pilot studies over a 6-year period and provided mentoring and support resources for young faculty investigators across multiple disciplines (see Table 8.1). Furthermore, we evaluated and refined our pilot studies program over time so that it more explicitly promoted community–researcher partnerships.

We worked closely during the first 3 years of CITRA with community partners to focus the CITRA pilot studies program on investigator development in the context of research in cooperation with community service agencies. Following the principles of partnership building in participatory research models (e.g., Israel et al., 1998), we organized volunteers from the CAC as a Pilot Studies Advisory Subcommittee. The committee's advice was essential for all phases of the program, including the development of the request for proposals (Wethington et al., 2007). A review committee consisting of both researchers and practitioners (who were recruited by the Pilot Studies Advisory Subcommittee) evaluated and rated the proposals for funding based on community responsiveness and priorities as well as standard research quality measures.

TABLE 8.1
The CITRA Pilot Studies Program: Selected Topics, Disciplines
of Investigators, and Community Partners

Year, no. of pilots funded	Research topics (selected)	Disciplines of pilot investigators	Community partners
Year 1, five pilots	Depression Pain Doctor–patient communication	Psychiatry Sociology Medicine	Health centers Home health agencies
Year 2, four pilots	Home-delivered meal recipients End of life care	Nutrition Medicine Psychology	Community service agencies Senior centers Case managers
Year 3, three pilots	Aging artists Elder self-neglect Depression care	Medicine Sociology Policy Analysis	Professional organizations Private foundations Senior centers Other universities
Year 4, three pilots	Life review Social isolation Health decision making	Psychiatry Psychology Economics	Senior centers Outpatient facilities
Year 5, two pilots	Chronic pain Health decision making	Psychology	Senior centers Home health care services
Year 6, four pilots	Consumer drug choices Social isolation and pain Prodomal symptoms of Alzheimer's disease	Linguistics Economics Psychology Psychiatry	Senior centers Home health care services Senior centers Other universities Outpatient facilities

We encouraged our investigators to adopt research implementation techniques from participatory research methods such as codeveloping research protocols with input from agencies hosting their research activities (see Israel et al., 1998; see also Chapter 2, this volume). This focus was consistent with our aim of providing the infrastructure to help develop projects with the capacity for translation to community practice. Some pilots incorporated a few techniques from participatory research models, and others evolved (with additional funding from other sources) as multiyear projects that involved community partners in development, implementation, analysis, and dissemination. It is most accurate to say that we expected our pilot investigators to adopt a participatory orientation (Minkler & Wallerstein, 2003), adopting principles appropriate to the aim of their pilot study. Thus, a pilot study could consist entirely of conducting focus groups with senior center clients and analyzing the data from the focus groups in partnership with agency and other stakeholders. In every case, however, pilot investigators were expected to use the pilot data for future proposal submissions or to develop larger projects that were informed by community input in their inception stages.

A condition of receipt of pilot studies funding was that the project apply to at least one part of the translational continuum (see Introduction, this volume). The projects we funded were all on the right side of the translational continuum (T2–T3), which was consistent with our mission. All projects involved the translation of social and behavioral science to a practical issue, such as pain management or end-of-life care. Two thirds of the pilots involved joint participation by a Cornell researcher and at least one community agency in New York City (the remaining one third were collaborations with health centers that had community outreach, except for two that were applied secondary analysis projects to develop data for future projects). We provided ongoing support to the investigator in developing a successful partnership. This included technical support to research investigators through CITRA's methodology core and the monthly work-in-progress seminars, and supervision and advice about the partnership development process. We also paid expenses for several researchers to travel to New York to develop a collaborative relationship with a community agency in preparation for submitting a proposal.

CITRA's pilot studies were successful both in providing service to agencies and in generating additional support for the researchers. A CITRA pilot study to improve treatment of geriatric depression in home health care served as pilot data for two successful NIH proposals (Sirey, 2008; Sirey, Raue, & Alexopoulous, 2007). Another pilot study to speed translation of nondrug therapies for older adults with chronic pain into practice settings led to a new NIH-funded behavioral intervention for use by community-dwelling older adults and eventual application through senior centers (Townley et al., 2010). A third was an interdisciplinary (psychology and economics) study of health decision making (Mikels, Reed, & Simon, 2009), which helped to secure National Science Foundation funding for the investigator and led to applications in Medicare Part D education programs.

The CITRA pilot studies program also sponsored the first study to document comprehensive data about the range of abilities and needs of 17,000 frail older people in New York City who receive home-delivered meals. The project was the first of many suggested by our community partners in response to changes being made in meal delivery. The research project, which interviewed recipients of 1,500 home-delivered meals in all five boroughs, was carried out in close collaboration with Citymeals, an agency that provides weekend meals for homebound older people (Frongillo, Cantor, et al., 2010;

Frongillo, Isaacman, Horan, Wethington, & Pillemer, 2010). CITRA investigators and the agency helped raise additional funds to support the project and conduct a follow-up with a subset of participants. The findings of the study led to modifications in home-delivered meals and a longer-term partnership with the agency. The agency, moreover, continues to collaborate with the Roybal Center on other pilot studies.

Two major emphases in our pilot studies program (and a focus of the proposal that created CITRA) were the development of innovative health survey methods for use in the field (this was a theme that had been established in the first 10 years of the Cornell Roybal Center) and a focus on health disparities among older people. *Disparities* were defined as differences between racial and ethnic groups in the incidence, prevalence, and burden of health conditions and disease (National Cancer Institute, 2010). Among the motives for partnering with investigators based in New York City in the renewal of the Roybal Center were to increase access of investigators based in Ithaca to racially and ethnically diverse populations and to address questions of great importance to the national health research enterprise (Smedley, Stith, & Nelson, 2003).

Addressing the needs of New York's diverse older population and addressing disparities in their health conditions and access to care also emerged as priorities during the initial community needs assessment and thus influenced the development of CITRA projects. For example, one pilot study assessed end-of-life preferences among older East Asians using qualitative methods (Rao, Desphande, Jamoona, & Reid, 2008). Another study used concept mapping as a way to identify factors associated with self-neglect among older people (not tending to one's hygiene and other basic needs) and to test the feasibility, reliability, and validity of the Cornell Scale for Self-Neglect (developed by the investigator), a tool for detecting and assessing the severity of such behaviors (Pavlou & Lachs, 2006, 2008). A secondary aim was to develop strategies for recruiting self-neglecters into research studies, a group that often avoids contact with others. A fourth methodologically innovative project conducted the first service needs assessment for aging artists in the New York metropolitan area (Jeffri, Heckathorn, & Spiller, 2011).

INVESTIGATOR DEVELOPMENT AND TRAINING

The monthly work-in-progress seminar was the focus of investigator development efforts. The aim of the seminar was to offer a mock "study section" for those who planned to submit proposals related to translational work on aging. In each seminar, two to three items were reviewed and critiqued, including grant proposals, articles, research protocols, study designs, and questionnaires. All affiliates were welcome to submit projects for critique.

The work-in-progress seminar also heard regularly scheduled reports from pilot investigators and preliminary presentations from investigators planning to submit pilot proposals. Pilot investigators were asked to bring problems or issues that had developed in their field work to the seminar for discussion. In this way, investigators were given feedback on how to solve small problems before they became big problems and how to address different aspects of the partnership. Monitoring of partnerships and sharing of expertise proved to be a highly efficient way of connecting with researchers; researchers and faculty affiliates considered the work in progress seminars to be the most useful of the activities offered to them by CITRA.

In addition to the seminars, core CITRA investigators mentored young investigators in proposal submissions. Over the 6-year period of the project, center investigators reviewed several dozen proposals submitted by pilot investigators and other faculty affiliates (potential pilot investigators). The training resources of the pilot program were also augmented by an Interdisciplinary Geriatrics Research Center grant from the Hartford Foundation under the management of the RAND Corporation. The grant funded several other pilots and provided additional education in interdisciplinary translational research for young investigators affiliated with CITRA.

The Hartford Foundation also funded the development of a new seminar on community-based scientific research on aging and health disparities, offered as a videoconference between Ithaca and New York City. The course continues between the two campuses of Cornell; participants have included pilot grantees, more experienced investigators, community partners, graduate students, postdoctoral researchers, fellows in geriatric medicine, and other medical students and trainees. The seminar is taught by former CITRA investigators and pilot grantees. It is the only course offered at Weill Cornell Medical College that teaches the principles of community-based participatory research and related methods and has become part of the Weill clinical and translational science master's program and the PhD program in human development at Cornell University in Ithaca.

FACILITATION OF RESEARCHER–PRACTITIONER INTERACTION

One indicator of the success of CITRA is that CAC partners requested participation from CITRA faculty and researchers in their activities and sought CITRA as a cosponsor for community events. These activities informed community agencies about the benefits of research, concepts of evidence-based practice, and similar issues. They also served as a means of developing community input for projects unrelated to CITRA, such as those developed by the Weill Clinical and Translational Science Center (founded in 2007). These projects fostered goodwill and built community capacity for collaborating with researchers (see also Stockdale, Mendel, Jones, Arroyo, & Gilmore, 2006). They also contributed to sustaining the "two-way" partnership between researchers and the community, wherein each group offered services of value to the other.

For example, CITRA cosponsored two workshops with CSCS on using the Internet to find evidence-based programs for implementation in centers. Based on one of its successful pilot projects, CITRA also cosponsored two trainings with the Geriatric Mental Health Alliance of New York and the New York State Department of Health on problem-solving therapy, an evidence-based clinical intervention for use with depressed older persons. CITRA investigators and affiliates were asked to speak at and participate in numerous other conferences and community events on topics such as research on social isolation among community-dwelling older people, food insecurity and older persons, the prevention of elder abuse, and new models for delivering senior center services. CITRA directors have also made presentations about partnership successes to community agencies and at the annual conference of CSCS. In addition, CITRA has made it possible for practitioners to address research audiences at Weill Cornell Medical College, providing an invaluable perspective that helps inform research priorities. (As previously mentioned, community partners sometimes attended the work-in-progress seminars and presented at the class on community-based research methods.)

The research-readiness and partnership building efforts paid dividends relatively early for CITRA. Under the direction of Cary Reid, we initiated a program of research to develop improved interventions to address the problem of chronic pain among older persons. Evidence-based treatments for chronic pain in the form of self-management programs have been developed for use in the community, and have demonstrated efficacy, but have been underutilized by older pain sufferers (Reid et al., 2008). Numerous barriers exist at the individual, program, and cultural levels that have a negative impact on program utilization, and these barriers need characterization to improve intervention strategies. Cornell researchers partnered with key stakeholders in New York City to build a community partnership focused on management of chronic pain. Two grants were funded by the NIH to develop innovative intervention protocols utilizing community input on development, implementation, and evaluation of evidence-based treatments for chronic pain. This project emerged from key priorities set by CITRA's CAC (managing impairments), as well as from the investigator's academic research interests. Other activities included the creation of a Chronic Pain Task Force in New York City to advise on setting the future research agenda and a conference on participatory research approaches to understanding pain, which took place in fall 2006 and was attended by nearly 100 practitioners.

RESEARCH-TO-PRACTICE CONSENSUS WORKSHOPS

A substantial amount of effort was devoted in the third year of CITRA to the development and testing of a model for bridging the gap between research-based knowledge and practice-based insight through the use of the consensus workshop model (defined below). The CITRA research-to-practice consensus workshop model (Sabir et al., 2006) was designed for two functions: (a) bringing research to practitioners in a setting in which they can learn about existing empirical research findings and (b) generating practice-based suggestions for new research directions that are responsive to the concerns of practitioners and their clients. The goal of this model is to create a two-way conversation between researchers and practitioners from which emerges a joint conception of an aging-related problem and the research that can help inform solutions for the problem. A recognized barrier in translational research is lack of understanding between researchers and practitioners, who take different approaches toward investigating and solving problems (see Young & Borland, 2011, for another approach). The model, which is described in greater detail elsewhere (Sabir et al., 2006), is briefly outlined here.

The CAC was responsible for selecting a list of topics for potential consensus workshops. The topics were then jointly selected for further development by the CITRA investigators and the CAC, based on five criteria: (a) a body of empirical research on the topic must already exist so that research can be reviewed; (b) the topic must be relevant to practice; (c) preferably, the topic must also be relevant to policy; (d) the topic must be relevant to what the community sees as a need; and (e) the review must not duplicate another recent and similar effort. The first topic selected for a consensus workshop was fall prevention among community-dwelling older persons. The second topic selected was social isolation among older adults, and later topics included elder abuse, persistent pain, and care transitions (e.g., Pillemer et al., 2011; Sabir et al., 2009).

For each topic, three community experts working in the area of interest were selected to aid in the review. In addition, three scientific research experts were selected to take part. The roles of the community and scientific research experts were (a) to provide consultation and guidance about existing research and major research questions; (b) to review drafts of the research review paper to be provided to workshop participants; (c) to help develop practice and policy recommendations; and (d) to attend the consensus workshop, bringing their own experiences and expertise to a discussion of the topic.

For each consensus workshop, a literature review of randomized controlled trials (RCTs) was conducted. We chose to introduce the findings from RCTs to CITRA's community partners to encourage further effectiveness studies in real-world community settings. (In areas where there were an insufficient number of published RCTs, we summarized research of the best scientific quality available.) This effort arose from our intentions to support practitioner understanding of research methods and to encourage rigorous evaluation of community-based programs. The literature was summarized in nontechnical language and sent to community practitioner experts, scientific research experts, and workshop participants. The consensus workshop, based on this document, was held, and researchers, practitioners, and community stakeholders discussed the document and set priorities for research studies. Recommendations of the workshop were widely disseminated to practitioners through our community partner CSCS, through the CITRA website, and in academic articles (e.g., Sabir et al., 2009). In several instances, CITRA funded pilot investigators to conduct studies to address issues raised in the consensus workshops.

THINGS WE WISH WE HAD DONE

Despite our achievements during the development of CITRA between 2003 and 2009, we wish we could have addressed important partnership and other activities in more depth. These activities were (a) formal evaluation of our dissemination activities, (b) research on implementation models in the community and whether the participatory process in which we engaged had an impact on the success of implementation, and (c) CITRA's potential impact on policy. We were a relatively small group of investigators and staff and had to use our time strategically, and thus we tended to build on successes that we had early in CITRA rather than break new ground in other areas. Our information about the impact of our dissemination efforts is anecdotal. We are acutely aware that little empirical evidence demonstrates that academic–community participatory models increase the impact of intervention programs and other research studies (Wallerstein & Duran, 2010). Finally, we lacked the methods for tracking our possible impact on policy and programs for older adults in New York City.

We also were never able to fully address some partnership issues within CITRA. The supply of investigators with the time and the inclination to conduct research in partnership with the community proved to be limited. Many researchers were willing to affiliate, but not all of them had research interests that matched needs identified in the community. Others were busy with projects and could not take the time to develop a new project. We received many more preliminary proposals for collaboration from the community than from researchers, and, often, worthy proposals from the community could not be matched to a researcher to carry them forward as a research study. This resulted from the fact that community agencies sometimes submitted requests for evaluation of existing programs rather than requests to develop new programs; the latter ideas are more likely to attract researchers. A more common reason was that researchers were already very busy and as a consequence were interested only in projects that fit logically with programs they had under way.

In contrast, it was much easier to find community partners for researchers who had ideas for research studies. Some of this mismatch may have resulted from our "let a thousand flowers bloom" philosophy, which encouraged community practitioners and researchers to address any topic relevant to social integration and isolation among aging people and the priorities laid out in the initial community needs assessment. In the current Cornell Roybal Center (2009 renewal) we addressed this problem partially by focusing on one area of research, managing chronic pain among older adults. This has made the balance of successfully resolved inquiries more equal in the partnership. But it has had its costs: The community partnership has also narrowed in focus and numbers.

LESSONS LEARNED AND CONCLUSION

We learned a number of lessons from the development of the CITRA partnership. First, it is essential to develop partnerships across levels, professions, and disciplines to provide the support investigators need in conducting translational research that has a practical impact on the health of communities. The CITRA investigators were too small a group to support every project; we constantly recruited research collaborators, such as health economists, experts on housing and community development, and research methodologists, to advise pilot mentees and develop grant proposals from the pilots. Similarly, we continually expanded our community contacts in New York City to find partners with the capacity to collaborate with research projects.

The second lesson we learned was that the partnership depended on its ability both to attract investigators and to engage practitioners and other potential community collaborators. Investigator development and education were necessary to bring research projects to fruition (see also Horowitz et al., 2009). The partnership required considerable nurturing on the academic side.

Third, we learned that the partnership had to be productive in the conventional research sense—papers published and proposals funded— to be supported by the collaborating academic and medical centers in the partnership. Institutional support is critical for sustaining community-researcher partnerships. We were fortunate that the research productivity of CITRA was recognized and that its investigator development activities were formally institutionalized by both campuses as credit-awarding classes. We were also fortunate to have a reservoir of faculty committed to applying research to real-world problems through their associations with Cornell Cooperative Extension and other outreach programs in the university.

To put these lessons into practice, we recommend that other partnerships among social and behavioral scientists, medical scientists, and the community start by building on existing strengths. We were lucky to have research and community relationships already in place that we could develop into an infrastructure that was ultimately larger than the sum of its parts. It was also ready to be implemented at the time of funding and thus required a shorter start-up period (it was "shovel-ready"), which is crucial for research productivity. We also recommend that the partnership be built with skilled and effective people who have experience working with communities and nonacademic audiences. We benefited from having assistant directors who had experience with community engagement through Cooperative Extension and other university outreach programs.

We recommend that the same care in selecting research and dissemination specialists also be applied when building a coalition of community partners. The initial community members of a partnership must have the capacity to engage in research and the motivation to do so. Building more extensive community capacity can be a goal of the partnership, but it is important to start with those agencies and groups that have the time, staffing, and experience to contribute to a partnership.

A third recommendation is to provide investigators with services and support that make it worth their while to work in partnership with the community. Even after recruiting investigators, we discovered that we had to continue investing time and mentorship to keep projects on track and to engage investigators beyond their initial pilot study funding. Developing partner-based research is a time-consuming activity for project directors, but it pays off in terms of productivity. The monthly work-in-progress seminar, regular contact with pilot investigators to check in on progress, and CITRA investigator mentorship of grant proposals were the three key activities.

A final recommendation is based on what we wish we had done: evaluate partnership activities, their reach to intended audiences, and their impact on the community using a formal model. In retrospect, we believe that our success would have been augmented by using formal evaluation principles to keep track of our impact on the community and on our institution, such as the RE-AIM model—reach, effectiveness, adoption, implementation, and maintenance (Glasgow, Vogt, & Boles, 1999). For example, it would have been useful to have kept track of the number of the agencies that felt they benefited from taking part in the partnership activities, whether other agencies were motivated to contact CITRA because of its programs, whether findings from the pilot projects were used to develop new programs at the agency level, and whether participating agencies were ready to partner again on additional research projects. (Anecdotally, we have heard from many of our community collaborators that they felt they benefited, and a number of centers and agencies have continued to collaborate with us.) It would also have been useful to follow up with our pilot investigators and determine whether they have continued to adopt participatory research principles in their studies. We do know that 75% of our pilot investigators were successful in obtaining additional funding to carry forward their projects and that their overall research productivity was higher (in terms of papers published per pilot study) than in the first 10 years of our Roybal Center (1993–2002). Formal evaluation of partnership models and their impact on both communities and researchers will be a task for the future in our Roybal Center.

REFERENCES

Drolet, B. C., & Lorenzi, N. M. (2011). Translating research: Understanding the continuum from bench to bedside. *Translational Research, 157*, 1–5. doi:10.1016/j.trsl.2010.10.002

Frongillo, E. A., Cantor, M. H., MacMillan, T., Issacman, T. D., Sherrow, R., Henry, M., . . . Pillemer, K. (2010). Who are the recipients of Meals-on-Wheels in New York City? A profile based on a representative sample of Meals-on-Wheels recipients, Part 1. *Care Management Journals, Journal of Long Term Home Health Care, 11*, 19–40. doi:10.1891/1521-0987.11.1.19

Frongillo, E. A., Isaacman, T. D., Horan, C. M., Wethington, E., & Pillemer, K. (2010). Adequacy of and satisfaction with delivery and use of home-delivered meals. *Journal of Nutrition for the Elderly, 29*, 211–226. doi:10.1080/01639361003772525

Glasgow, R. E., Vogt, T. M., & Boles, S. M. (1999). The public health impact of health promotion interventions: The RE-AIM framework. *American Journal of Public Health, 89*, 1322–1327. doi:10.2105/AJPH.89.9.1322

Horowitz, C. R., Robinson, M., & Seifer, S. (2009). Community-based participatory research from the margin to the mainstream: Are researchers prepared? *Circulation, 19*, 2633–2642. doi:10.1161/CIRCULATIONAHA.107.729863

Israel, B. A., Schulz, A. J., Parker, E. A., & Becker, A. B. (1998). Review of community-based participatory research: Assessing partnership approaches to improve public health. *Annual Review of Public Health, 19*, 173–202. doi:10.1146/annurev.publhealth.19.1.173

Jeffri, J., Heckathorn, D. D., & Spiller, M. W. (2011). Painting your life: A study of aging visual artists in New York City. *Poetics, 39*(1), 19–43. doi:10.1016/j.poetic.2010.11.001

Jones, L., & Wells, K. (2007). Strategies for academic and clinical engagement in community-participatory partnered research. *JAMA*, *297*, 407–410. doi:10.1001/jama.297.4.407

Khoury, M. J., Gwinn, M., Yoon, P. W., Dowling, N., Moore, C. A., & Bradley, L. (2007). The continuum of translation research in genomic medicine: How can we accelerate the appropriate integration of human genome discoveries into health care and disease prevention? *Genetics in Medicine*, *9*, 665–674. doi:10.1097/GIM.0b013e31815699d0

Mikels, J. A., Reed, A. E., & Simon, K. I. (2009). Older adults place lower value on choice relative to younger adults. *Journals of Gerontology: Series B: Psychological Sciences and Social Sciences*, *64B*, 443–446. doi:10.1093/geronb/gbp021

Minkler, M., & Wallerstein, N. (2003). Introduction to community-based participatory research. In M. Minkler & N. Wallerstein (Eds.), *Community-based participatory research for health* (pp. 4–26). San Francisco, CA: Jossey-Bass.

National Cancer Institute. (2010). *Health disparities defined*. Retrieved from http://crchd.cancer.gov/disparities/defined.html

National Council on Aging. (2006). *Using the evidence base to promote healthy aging: The Administration on Aging's Evidence-Based Prevention Programs for the Elderly Initiative*. Washington, DC: National Council on Aging.

Office of Behavioral and Social Sciences Research. (2007). *The contribution of the behavioral and social sciences research to improving the health of the nation: A prospectus for the future*. Bethesda, MD: National Institutes of Health.

Pavlou, M. P., & Lachs, M. S. (2006). Could self-neglect in older adults be a geriatric syndrome? *Journal of the American Geriatrics Society*, *54*, 831–842. doi:10.1111/j.1532-5415.2006.00661.x

Pavlou, M. P., & Lachs, M. S. (2008). Self-neglect in older adults: A primer for clinicians. *Journal of General Internal Medicine*, *23*, 1841–1846. doi:10.1007/s11606-008-0717-7

Pillemer, K., Breckman, R., Sweeney, C. D., Brownell, P., Fulmer, T., Bernan, J., . . . Lachs, M. S. (2011). Practitioners' views on elder mistreatment research priorities: Recommendations from a research-to-practice conference. *Journal of Elder Abuse & Neglect*, *23*, 115–126. doi:10.1080/08946566.2011.558777

Pillemer, K., Czaja, S., Schulz, R., & Stahl, S. (2003). Finding the best ways to help: Opportunities and challenges of intervention research on aging. *The Gerontologist*, *43*, 5–8. doi:10.1093/geront/43.suppl_1.5

Pillemer, K., Moen, P., Wethington, E., & Glasgow, N. (Eds.). (2000). *Social integration in the second half of life*. Baltimore, MD: Johns Hopkins University Press.

Pillemer, K., Suitor, J. J., & Wethington, E. (2003). Integrating theory, basic research, and intervention: Examples from caregiving research. *The Gerontologist*, *43*, 19–28. doi:10.1093/geront/43.suppl_1.19

Rao, A. S., Desphande, O. M., Jamoona, C., & Reid, M. C. (2008). Elderly Indo-Caribbean Hindus and end-of-life care: A community-based exploratory study. *Journal of the American Geriatrics Society, 56,* 1129–1133. doi:10.1111/j.1532-5415.2008.01723.x

Reid, M. C., Papaleontiou, M., Ong, A., Breckman, R., Wethington, E., & Pillemer, K. (2008). Self-management strategies to reduce pain and improve functions among older adults in community settings: A review of the evidence. *Pain Medicine, 9,* 409–424. doi:10.1111/j.1526-4637.2008.00428.x

Sabir, M., Breckman, R., Meador, R., Wethington, E., Reid, M. C., & Pillemer, K. (2006). The CITRA Research–Practice Consensus–Workshop Model: Exploring a new method of research translation in aging. *The Gerontologist, 46,* 833–839. doi:10.1093/geront/46.6.833

Sabir, M., Wethington, E., Breckman, R., Meador, R., Reid, M. C., & Pillemer, K. (2009). A community-based participatory critique of social isolation intervention research for community-dwelling older adults. *Journal of Applied Gerontology, 28,* 218–234. doi:10.1177/0733464808326004

Sirey, J. A. (2008). The impact of psychosocial factors on experience of illness and mental health service use. *American Journal of Geriatric Psychiatry, 16,* 703–705. doi:10.1097/JGP.0b013e318182550b

Sirey, J. A., Raue, P. J., & Alexopoulos, G. S. (2007). An intervention to improve depression care in older adults with COPD. *International Journal of Geriatric Psychiatry, 22,* 154–159. doi:10.1002/gps.1705

Smedley, B. D., Stith, A. Y., & Nelson, A. R. (Eds.) 2003. *Unequal treatment: Confronting racial and ethnic disparities in health care.* Committee on Understanding Racial and Ethnic Disparities in Health Care, Board of Health Sciences Policy, Institute of Medicine. Washington, DC: National Academies Press.

Stockdale, S. E., Mendel, P., Jones, J., Arroyo, W., & Gilmore, J. (2006). Assessing organizational readiness and change in community intervention research: Framework for participatory evaluation. *Ethnicity & Disease, 16,* S1-136–S1-145.

Townley, S., Papaleontiou, M., Amanfo, L., Henderson, C., Pillemer, K., Beissner, K., & Reid, M. C. (2010). Preparing to implement a self-management program for back pain in New York City senior centers: What do prospective clients think? *Pain Medicine, 11,* 405–415. doi:10.1111/j.1526-4637.2009.00783.x

Trochim, W., & Kane, M. (2005). Concept mapping: An introduction to structured conceptualization in health care. *International Journal for Quality in Health Care, 17,* 187–191. doi:10.1093/intqhc/mzi038

Wallerstein, N., & Duran, B. (2010). Community-based participatory research contributions to intervention research: The intersection of science and practice to improve health equity. *American Journal of Public Health, 100,* S40–S46. doi:10.2105/AJPH.2009.184036

Westfall, J. M., Mold, J., & Fagnan, L. (2007). Practice-based research—"blue highways" on the NIH Roadmap. *JAMA, 297,* 403–406. doi:10.1001/jama.297.4.403

Wethington, E., Breckman, R., Meador, R., Lachs, M. S., Reid, M. C., Sabir, M., & Pillemer, K. (2007). The CITRA pilot studies program: Mentoring translational research. *The Gerontologist, 47,* 845–850. doi:10.1093/geront/47.6.845

Wethington, E., & Pillemer, K. (2007, Winter). Translating basic research into community practice: The Cornell Institute for Translational Research on Aging (CITRA). *Forum on Public Policy Online.* Available at http://www.forumonpublicpolicy.com

Young, D., & Borland, R. (2011). Conceptual challenges in the translation of research into practice: It's not just a matter of "communication." *Translational Behavioral Medicine, 1*(2), 256–269. doi:10.1007/s13142-011-0035-1

AFTERWORD

RACHEL E. DUNIFON AND ELAINE WETHINGTON

This volume presents models and examples of social and behavioral science–based translational research. We use a definition of *translational research* that would likely please our inspiration, Urie Bronfenbrenner: the linkage of theoretically driven basic research to understanding interventions or policies that improve human health and well-being, evaluation of interventions or policies for efficacy and effectiveness, and application of field experience to future development of basic theory and its applications (Pillemer, Suitor, & Wethington, 2003, p. 20). As this definition makes clear, social and behavioral scientists have key roles to play in translational research. This volume highlights the benefits to scholars who take part in translational research, as well as the challenges and complexities inherent in engaging in translational research.

These complexities emerged at the 2009 Biennial Urie Bronfenbrenner Conference, which was the catalyst for this book, and are expanded upon in this volume. The work in this book has presented several social and behavioral science models for the translation of research, followed by case studies of translation of basic social and behavioral sciences into projects aimed at improving health, quality of life, and professional practice. In this Afterword, we comment on models for translational research in the social and behavioral sciences, barriers to conducting translational research, how these barriers can be reduced, and opportunities for interested social and behavioral scientists to take part in the research translation.

MODELS FOR TRANSLATIONAL RESEARCH IN THE SOCIAL AND BEHAVIORAL SCIENCES

Three types of models for social and behavioral science–based translational research have emerged in the book: (a) researcher–consumer interaction in developing research questions and in partnering on dissemination into professional practice networks; (b) qualitative–quantitative mixed model approaches to enhance communication between researcher and practitioner groups; and (c) community participatory research methods that engage local organizations in the conduct of research studies to raise awareness of research, to emphasize the need for evaluation, and to promote the use of evidence-based practices.

Several authors identified the importance of listening to the consumers of social and behavioral science research—the policymakers and practitioners for whom scholarly research is relevant. As noted by Wandersman and Lesesne (Chapter 2), doing so allows for consumer input into the very questions that researchers ask, with the end result benefiting both researchers and consumers. The importance of listening to consumers is a key factor in the Interactive Systems Framework of Wandersman and Lesesne and emerged in several of the case studies. For example, Crosnoe (Chapter 3) highlighted his own transformation as a scholar, in which he discovered the benefits of communicating with the consumers of his research, in this case local school district officials. Such communication helped him identify key research questions, leading to work that was not only rewarding from a research perspective but that also, because it was designed with the input of policymakers up front, could address important real-world questions. Ispa (Chapter 5) and Almeida and coauthors (Chapter 6) related similar stories of the benefits of communicating with consumers at the inception of a research project. In Ispa's case, this was the director of the local Early Head Start program. In the case of Almeida and colleagues, researchers worked with partners in the hotel industry who helped them identify the questions to be examined and translate the results of their work back into the industry for wider dissemination. Similarly, the investigators of the Cornell Institute for Translational Research on Aging (CITRA; Chapter 8) created a partnership for facilitating input into policies affecting service delivery to older people in New York City and disseminating evidence-based practices through existing service professional networks.

Several papers focused on the benefits of employing mixed qualitative–quantitative approaches when conducting social and behavioral science–based translational research. As noted by both Crosnoe and Ispa, such methods give voice to those who are most directly influenced by the policy, program, or condition being studied. These methods add more nuanced knowledge to a research study and provide a strong set of tools that researchers can use to communicate with the end consumers of the research. Although it may be a source of frustration that policymakers and practitioners find a single anecdote more compelling than a multifaceted regression-based analysis, mixed methods research provides translational scholars with a way to make this work to their advantage.

Other papers focused on community participatory methods, among which community-based participatory research (CBPR) is the most prominent (Chapters 1, 4, and 8). Participatory models engage relevant community organizations such as social service agencies, health advocates, and churches in all aspects of a research study. Partnering with local organizations to engage minority communities in research may be key because trust in public institutions may be low these communities (Jones & Wells, 2007). Partnering with the community increases access to local knowledge about the problems to be addressed, which assists in planning for the types of interventions that will be effective and increases the capacity of the community to sustain the intervention after the research has been completed. Participatory models have the potential to close the gap between research findings and their application in real-world settings.

BARRIERS TO CONDUCTING TRANSLATIONAL RESEARCH IN THE SOCIAL AND BEHAVIORAL SCIENCES

The chapters in this volume also discussed some of the barriers to conducting social and behavioral science–based translational research. First, as noted by Wethington, Herman, and Pillemer in the Introduction, the term *translational research* has, for the most part, been defined by the biomedical field. Even in performing what using our definition would be called translational research, social and behavioral scientists often do not use the term. As a case in point, prior to the 2009 Bronfenbrenner Conference, Pillemer and Wethington conducted an extensive review of 224 articles on translational research covering the years 1999–2007. They found only about 50 articles in psychology, sociology, gerontology, and public health journals that used the term *translational research* in their titles. Perlstadt (2009), reviewing articles in the mainstream sociology journals for 1990–2009, found only two articles that used the term *translational research* in their text. In addition, the 60 clinical and translational centers funded by the National Institutes of Health (NIH) are the public face of translational research in the United States, and many do not include social and behavioral scientists in their leadership teams. (One notable exceptions, the leadership team at the Weill Cornell Medical College in New York City, includes a psychologist as the head of evaluation.) The NIH Clinical and Translational Science Awards initiative, and by implication translational research, is viewed as focusing on biomedical rather than behavioral research (Breckler, 2008).

In addition, as noted by both Crosnoe and Ispa, the social and behavioral science academic community often does not value the time-consuming, multimethod, iterative nature of translational research. Social and behavioral scientists may often lack the training necessary to conduct translational research as well. This includes a lack of training in how to develop partnerships with the community and a lack of training in the methods noted above, specifically mixed method and community participatory approaches to research (e.g., Horowitz, Robinson, & Seifer, 2009).

REDUCING BARRIERS TO TRANSLATIONAL RESEARCH

As shown throughout this volume, these barriers are slowly eroding. Crosnoe discussed how his work as a translational scholar was transformed through unique and innovative funding mechanisms such as the William T. Grant Foundation Scholars Program, the Foundation for Child Development Changing Faces of America's Youth early career program, and the Eunice Kennedy Shriver National Institute of Child Health and Human Development (NICHD) Early Child Care Research Network. Each of these groups explicitly promoted interdisciplinary, multimethod applied research activities that fostered Crosnoe's development as a translational scholar. Indeed, as Evans made clear in Chapter 1, NIH has put forth a series of innovative requests for proposals and program announcements in recent years, seeking to promote and broaden the scope of translational research in ways that facilitate the involvement of social and behavioral scientists. Further examples include Ispa's work with the Early Head Start Research Consortium, in which the project's funding mandated that the team conduct research that was explicitly translational in nature—research that would be immediately used to improve the program and that was informed by the team's community partners. As Ispa noted, Urie Bronfenbrenner was key in building these translational components into the evaluation design and the request for proposals. Almeida and colleagues also highlighted the key role that innovative funding can play in promoting translational research, both from private foundations (the Alfred P. Sloan Foundation) and the federal government

(NICHD). Finally, Wethington, Pillemer, and Meador (Chapter 8) described the CITRA model, which grew out of a commitment by the National Institute on Aging to promote translational research on aging. As these examples make clear, funders are leading the way in transforming how the research community thinks about and conducts translational research.

The barriers to conducting translational research in the social and behavioral sciences can be further reduced. As the papers presented here show, translational research is often best done as part of a team. Crosnoe (Chapter 3), Ispa (Chapter 5), Almeida and colleagues (Chapter 6), and Wethington and colleagues (Chapter 8) discussed the benefits of a team-based approach to their translational research activities. As described here, translational research requires mixed methods, consumer input, and iterative feedback loops between research and policy or practice. This is certainly a tall order for a single researcher! Using a team-based approach reduces this burden, as different team members can contribute various methods and skills. If one conceives of translational research as a continuum of tasks as shown in Figure 1 of the Introduction to this volume (see also Drolet & Lorenzi, 2011), the team approach emerges clearly.

This volume makes clear that scholars doing translational research do not necessarily have to take on the process of translation to practice themselves. A focus on practical outcomes and influencing important institutions when selecting research questions also contributes to the overall enterprise of translational research. As shown by Zember and coauthors (Chapter 7), researchers can work through professional organizations to disseminate findings to practitioners. Furthermore, Crosnoe and Almeida and colleagues documented how successful community–researcher partnerships can facilitate the translation process: When consumers are brought into the process from the beginning, they have a greater stake in the ultimate findings and, in turn, are more invested in speeding the translation of those results back into their work. Wethington and colleagues in Chapter 8 described how they created a researcher–community partnership that placed researchers in roles that bring science to the community and community perspectives back to the science. People from both the research and the practice sides can benefit from education about how to work together by learning about each other's perspectives (points reiterated by Crosnoe and Wandersman and Lesesne in this volume).

Beyond the ways in which individual scholars approach their work, many activities can be engaged in by members of various academic disciplines to reduce the barriers to conducting social and behavioral science–based translational research. Educating young scholars about the methods and opportunities for translational research would be an important step. Crosnoe, in his chapter, described a series of more and less successful attempts to self-train as a translational scholar; such fits and starts could be reduced if translational research was incorporated into social and behavioral science training programs. In addition, research on the translational process itself is needed, as highlighted in Chapter 4 by Krivitsky and colleagues. Social and behavioral science fields would benefit from the presentation of more case studies showing challenges and successes for translational research.

FUTURE OPPORTUNITIES FOR TRANSLATIONAL RESEARCH IN THE SOCIAL AND BEHAVIORAL SCIENCES

As noted by Evans and by Wandersman and Lesesne, the current debates and policy changes in regard to health care reform present a unique opportunity for social and behavioral scientists to contribute through rigorous translational research. Beyond the health care debate, a variety of opportunities for social and behavioral science–based translational research exist. These opportunities include

- taking part in multi- and interdisciplinary structures that integrate university scientists and practitioners;
- developing the science of systematic research reviews to encourage reviews that are accessible and practical enough to be used by practitioners and policymakers as well as by researchers;
- developing and using rigorous intervention designs to test social and psychological contributions to healthy development (e.g., Cicchetti & Toth, 2009; Greenberg, 2006);
- contributing to effective and sustainable interventions in the community by applying social and behavioral science theories (e.g., Burgio, 2010);
- taking part in university community outreach to involve community organizations and representatives in setting research priorities;
- incorporating community input into smaller, individual research projects;
- conducting research on the translational process itself as a means of scientific innovation;
- conducting innovative research on the ultimate outcomes of the translational research process—the impact on public health and well-being; and
- incorporating demographic and other research that documents characteristics of communities, schools, and other locations in which policies and programs are taking place, thereby identifying areas of need for intervention as well as documenting trends in well-being that are related to changes in policy and practice.

CONCLUDING THOUGHTS

Overall, the future of translational research in the social and behavioral sciences is dependent on returning to our inspiration, Urie Bronfenbrenner, and taking his model to heart. This suggests that translational research scholars recognize and incorporate the multiple, interacting influences on our work from multiple disciplines, various methods, external consumer factors, and the larger political climate in which our work takes place.

At Cornell University we are fortunate to have a newly developed center devoted to addressing some of the challenges and opportunities noted here. The Bronfenbrenner Center for Translational Research (BCTR) in Cornell's College of Human Ecology will work to increase the capacity for translational research among Cornell faculty, researchers, and students by creating a "living laboratory" for the extension of research-based knowledge into practice and policy settings. The center's overarching goal is to create a seamless relationship between theory-driven, fundamental science on the one hand and application and innovation in real-world settings on the other. The BCTR will train scholars (including faculty and students) in translational research, support translational research programs, and provide opportunities for connection between researchers and the community. As such, the BCTR stands as an excellent example of the future of translational research in the social and behavioral sciences.

Engagement in the translation of basic social and behavioral research to human health and well-being is not only a worthy scientific endeavor— it is also a necessity in order to demonstrate the worth of federal and private investment in the social and behavioral research enterprise in a time of shrinking resources. Investment in social and behavioral science renders our disciplines—psychology, human development, sociology, demography, economics, gerontology—accountable to the public.

REFERENCES

Breckler, S. J. (2008). The NIH roadmap: Are psychologists in or out? *Journal of Clinical Psychology in Medical Settings, 15*(1), 60–64. doi:10.1007/s10880-008-9099-6

Burgio, L. D. (2010). Disentangling the translational sciences: A social science perspective. *Research and Theory for Nursing Practice, 24*(1), 56–63. doi:10.1891/1541-6577.24.1.56

Cicchetti, D., & Toth, S. L. (2009). The past achievements and future promises of developmental psychopathology: The coming of age of a discipline. *Journal of Child Psychology and Psychiatry, 50*(1–2), 16–25. doi:10.1111/j.1469-7610.2008.01979.x

Drolet, B. C., & Lorenzi, N. M. (2011). Translating research: Understanding the continuum from bench to bedside. *Translational Research, 157,* 1–5. doi:10.1016/j.trsl.2010.10.002

Greenberg, M. T. (2006). Promoting resilience in children and youth: Preventive interventions and their interface with neuroscience. *Annals of the New York Academy of Sciences, 1094,* 139–150. doi:10.1196/annals.1376.013

Horowitz, C. R., Robinson, M., & Seifer, S. (2009). Community-based participatory research from the margin to the mainstream: Are researchers prepared? *Circulation, 119,* 2633–2642. doi:10.1161/CIRCULATIONAHA.107.729863

Jones, L., & Wells, K. (2007). Strategies for academic and clinical engagement in community-participatory partnered research. *JAMA, 297,* 407–410. doi:10.1001/jama.297.4.407

Perlstadt, H. (2009). Translational research: Enabling the biomedical and social behavioral sciences to benefit society. *Humboldt Journal of Social Relations, 32*(1), 4–34.

Pillemer, K., Suitor, J. J., & Wethington, E. (2003). Integrating theory, basic research, and intervention: Two case studies from caregiving research. *The Gerontologist, 43*(Suppl. 1), 19–28. doi:10.1093/geront/43.suppl_1.19

INDEX

Early Head Start, 57, 105, 108–114,
    116–120
Early Head Start Research Consortium,
    105–107, 110, 117
EBPs. *See* Evidence-based practices
Economic forces, 55–56
Economics of Health Care Reform, 28
Educational and developmental
        research, 53–69
    cultural understanding in, 66–68
    and inequality in education system,
        54–59
    for large-scale vs. small-scale policy,
        62–63
    methodological approaches in,
        63–65
    and relationship with policymakers,
        65–66
    translational, 53–54, 59–62
Educational settings, 9
Edward R. Roybal Center for Transla-
        tional Research on Aging, 10, 170.
        See also Roybal Centers
Efficacy, 4
Emotion, secondhand, 138
Empirical evidence, 63–64
Employees
    hotel. *See* Hotel employees
    hourly, 131
Engagement, 48
Environment, social, 23
Environmental conditions, 104, 105
Ethical obligations, 117–119
Ethnically diverse communities, 4
Ethnographic data, 64–65
Eunice Kennedy Shriver National Insti-
        tute of Child Health and Human
        Development (NICHD), 24–25,
        132, 135, 141, 163
European American families, 114
Evaluation, formal, 90–91, 184
Evidence
    DNA, 151–152, 160–161
    empirical, 63–64
    given by children, 154–155
    infected with false memories,
        152–153
    legal, 148
    physical, 156–157
    scientific, 59

Evidence-Based Disease and Disability
        Prevention Program, 73
Evidence-based practices (EBPs)
    application of, 6–8
    diffusion of, 4, 73–74, 78–79
    for health and well-being, 4
    types of adaptations for, 81, 88–91
Exonerations, 160–161
Experts, 183
External validity, 27, 28, 35–37
Eyewitness identification, 150–153,
    157–161

Fagnan, L., 8, 40–41
False confessions, 150–153
False memory, 147–163
    in adults, 159–161
    in children, 156–159
    in confessions, 150–153
    in eyewitness identification, 150–153
    fuzzy trace theory of, 153–156
    in legal judgment and decision
        making, 161–162
    problems caused by, 147–150
False memory reports, 155
False-persistence effect, 155–156
False superiority, 156
Families. *See also* Parents; Work–family
        conflict
    African American, 108, 112
    emotional transmission in, 134–135
    European American, 114
    low-income, 105, 112
    parenting and education in, 57–58
    protection of, from false memories,
        149–150
    research on, 108
    and schools, 57–58
Federal policymakers, 62–63
Feedback, direct, 90
Feminist theory, 109
Fidelity, maintenance of, 92
Findings, 139–141
Fine, Mark, 107–109
Fischer, C. S., 55–56
Fiscian, V. S., 82
Flaspohler, P., 45
Flexibility, 110, 140
Focus on Kids, 74
Forensic science, 157

ABOUT THE EDITORS

Elaine Wethington, PhD, is professor of human development and of sociology at Cornell University, Ithaca. She is a specialist in the sociology of mental health, aging, and the life course. She received her PhD in sociology from the University of Michigan in 1987. Since 2003, she has been both the codirector of the Cornell–Columbia Edward R. Roybal Center for Translational Research on Aging and the director of its Pilot Studies Core (funded by the National Institute on Aging). She is also an associate director of the Bronfenbrenner Center for Translational Research. Dr. Wethington is the author of many papers on life stress and health, translational research on aging, health and the work–family interface, and life turning points. Currently, she is also the coprincipal investigator for Small Changes and Lasting Effects, an obesity behavioral intervention study funded by the National Heart, Lung, and Blood Institute (NHLBI); coinvestigator for a cohort study of life stress and heart disease (Novel Measures of Psychosocial Stress, funded by NHLBI); and coinvestigator for Nudging Nutrition: Setting Healthier Defaults in Supermarkets and Homes (funded by the National Institutes of Health, American Recovery and Reinvestment Act of 2009 Challenge Program).

Rachel E. Dunifon, PhD, is associate professor in the department of policy analysis and management at Cornell University. She received her PhD in human development and social policy from Northwestern University in 1999 and was a postdoctoral fellow at the University of Michigan's Poverty Research and Training Center. Her expertise is in the area of child and family policy, with a focus on how policy-relevant family factors influence child well-being. Her recent research focuses on maternal employment patterns, family functioning and child well-being, and the role of grandparents in the lives of children. Dr. Dunifon is also the associate director in Cornell's Bronfenbrenner Center for Translational Research and leads an outreach program called Parenting in Context, designed to use research-based information to inform parent education programs.